Surgical MCQ ..dates

Computer Typesetting by Print Origination Ltd.,
Hawthorne Road, Bootle, Merseyside, L20 6NS

Surgical MCQs for Undergraduates

J.L.Craven, B.Sc., M.D., F.R.C.S.
Consultant Surgeon,
York District Hospital;
Lately Senior Lecturer in Surgery,
Welsh National School of Medicine, Cardiff

J.S.P.Lumley, M.B., B.S., F.R.C.S.
Assistant Director, Surgical Unit, and
Honorary Consultant in Surgery,
St. Bartholomew's Hospital, London

CHURCHILL LIVINGSTONE
Edinburgh London and New York 1976

CHURCHILL LIVINGSTONE

Medical Division of Longman Group Limited

Distributed in the United States of
America by Longman Inc., 19 West 44th Street, New
York, N.Y. 10036 and by associated companies,
branches and representatives throughout the
world.

First edition 1976
  Reprinted 1978

ISBN 0 443 01463 9

Printed in Hong Kong by Wilture Enterprises (International) Ltd.

To Pauline and Jean

Preface

An examination system which is to assess the results of a number of years of study should do so fairly, uniformly and reliably, it should cover as much of the syllabus as possible, and be able to differentiate between good and bad candidates in a consistent manner. The objective test succeeds to a large degree in fulfilling these requirements but in itself it must not be a handicap to the candidate who should be well versed in this form of examination technique.

It is not claimed that the questions in the subsequent chapters will provide a painless method of passing the undergraduate's surgical finals, for it is hoped that the horizon of examining boards will include data obtained from other important spheres such as continuous assessment, long-term case studies, oral assessment and conventional essay-style questions. It is hoped that the book will provide the student with an introduction to objective testing and, in particular, with a method of both testing and improving his surgical knowledge.

We are grateful to Churchill Livingstone for the speedy and effective help they gave us in publishing this book.

April, 1976

J. L. Craven
J.S.P. Lumley

Introduction

Objective Testing

The perfect examination would be one in which the student was accurately assessed in his knowledge, comprehension, application, analysis and evaluation of material pertinent to the subject being examined. The use of the essay type question paper as the sole means of assessment has been criticised because of its reliance on subjective (and therefore unmeasurable) qualities.

For several years educationalists of many different disciplines have sought methods of objective testing which examined all the above mentioned qualities. In all objective tests the student has to choose the correct response out of one or more alternatives, his answers being either right or wrong. The subjective judgement of the examiner thus plays no part in this form of examination. Objective testing has been used extensively in the U.S.A. since the end of the Second World War, but introduction in the U.K. has been slow, and it has reached the universities generally via schools and technical colleges. However, a multiple choice question paper is now in use in most medical schools and it has been necessary for both the medical student and his teacher to become fully acquainted with the uses and abuses of this testing technique. It is appropriate here to consider the merits of the various examination techniques and, perhaps most important, to compare objective testing with the traditional essay question.

The Essay

Students and examiners have questioned the effectiveness of an essay paper in measuring the attainment of a number of years of study. The area covered by such an examination is very limited, the more so when a wide choice of questions is allowed. It thus encourages the students to 'spot questions' and to concentrate on only part of the syllabus. The marking of essays is time consuming and unreliable, there being marked variations in an individual examiner's reassessment of papers as well as between examiners. This variation makes comparison on a national level difficult and is further accentuated by what has been described as the deep psychological barrier of examiners to allocate more than seventy per cent of the total marks allowed for any given essay question. However the essay does determine the candidate's ability to write clear and legible English, it tests his ability to collect and quantitate material and it assesses his powers of logic, original thought and creativity. In terms of cost the essay question is cheap to produce but it is expensive to mark.

The Composition of Objective Questions

The objective form of examination is best composed by a panel of examiners, each having a complete understanding of the syllabus and a thorough knowledge of the field of study. The panel must first decide the parts of the syllabus to be covered by the examination, and the level of knowledge required by the candidate. The type of objective test and the number of options per question is decided and each member of the panel prepares a set of questions for the group to consider. A multiple choice question consists of a stem (the initial question) and four or more options; one of these options in the multiple choice question is correct and this is known as the key, the incorrect responses being known as the distractors. In the case of multiple response questions, there may be more than one correct response. (This form of question has also been termed multiple completion, multiple answer, multiple true or false and the indeterminate response by various authorities, but in most centres, and in this text, it will subsequently be referred to as a multiple choice question).

Stem and options should be brief using the minimum number of words and the instructions should be clear and simple, the language used being appropriate to the verbal ability and requirement of the candidate. The question must always be of some educational value. The words 'always' and 'never' should be avoided and the stem should preferably not be in the negative. There should be no recurrent phrase in the options which can be included in the stem. The key (the correct option or options) must be wholly correct and unambiguous. It is important for the correct response to be in different positions in each of a group of questions and some form of random allocation may be necessary. The distractors (the wrong options) are the most exacting and challenging part of objective question composition and the standard of an objective test is probably best assessed in terms of the quality of its distractors. They must always be plausible, yet completely wrong. They should be in a parallel style to the key and they should not contain clues. Common misconceptions form good distractors. 'None of them' or 'all of them' are not satisfactory distractors. Four options are thought by many authorities to be sufficient.

After the draft questions have been collected, it is advisable for a panel of examiners to assess their value and limitations. Inaccurate and irrelevant material is then excluded. Even the most experienced of examiners will find that a panel will offer constructive criticism on the majority of his questions. Ideally, once the panel has accepted a series of questions these should be pre-tested on a group of students and the results analysed. It is desirable for a question to have been pre-tested on 300 to 400 students before it comes into regular use in a qualifying examination. The difficulty of a question can be determined by calculating the percentage of students giving the right answer, and its discriminatory value (the ratio of correct/incorrect responses) calculated in a manner which takes into account whether or not the better students obtained the correct response. The facility value (difficulty index) records the percentage of correct responses and compares it with the total number of candidates. Additional information on the mean range of distribution of the answers can also be obtained with a discriminatory index and a bi-serial correlation coefficient (relating the total candidate response to an option, with the results of the top 27 per cent and the bottom 27 per cent of the candidates to the same option). Figures for both the discriminatory index and the bi-serial correlation coefficient range from plus 1 to minus 1. Questions with factors of less than 0.20 should be rejected (unless a few difficult or easy questions are to be included). Values of 0.21 to 0.29 are of marginal discriminatory value. The values 0.30 to 0.39 show a reasonable discriminatory power of the option, whereas results greater than 0.44 indicate good discrimination by a question of the candidates under test. The effectiveness of the question is also measured in terms of the number of students attempting it—the value of a question certainly cannot be assessed if a large number of students leave it out. Computer readouts on a series of questions will also provide the ranking of students, the scatter of the results and a raw score (i.e. the number of correct less the number of incorrect results).

The pre-testing, though very time consuming, greatly adds to the validity and reliability of the objective test. Using the results of these tests the panel can rephrase unsatisfactory questions and compile the definitive examination paper. The time allowed in the pre-test is not limited but the students are asked to note the time taken to complete the test; the time required for the final version is thus arrived at. This time should allow at least 90 per cent of the candidates to complete the paper. It is usual to start an examination paper with a few easier questions (i.e. with a low difficulty index) and similarly a few difficult questions can be included at the end. It has been found that a good (wide) range of results is obtained by setting a large number of questions with average discrimination rather then including a large number with high or low discriminatory indices. Testing of the questions should not stop after the pre-testing phase, the information gained from each subsequent examination should be used to continuously review all the question material.

Obviously a series of questions which have been pre-tested and shown to be satisfactory is of great value to the examiner. Such questions can be used repeatedly provided they have not been freely available to the student. Security is an important factor, particularly when the number of questions is small and does not cover the whole syllabus. For this reason it is advisable to have a large number of questions available. It is reasonable to assume that if a student is capable of memorising the correct responses to a large number of questions (even if these are known to him) he will also have a passable knowledge of the syllabus.

A satisfactory bank of questions takes three to five years to build. After this time the questions can be grouped into sections and, whenever an examination paper is required, questions can be chosen at random from each section. Continuous updating and revision of this material should be undertaken and new material added regularly. The history of each question in the bank should be recorded. Repetitive use of the questions over a number of years allows annual standards to be compared.

The Student's Approach To Objective Testing

Any student required to undertake an objective test for a qualifying examination or post-graduate examination should ensure he has some preliminary experience in this form of testing. It is essential for him to know and have sampled the style of questions used by his particular examining board.

In any objective test all the instructions provided must be carefully read and understood and the student's designated number marked in the appropriate section, otherwise a computer marking system will reject the paper—this will not impress the examining authority.

The type of objective test used in medical education does vary and some of these types have already been discussed. Whatever form the question takes in the objective test it is essential that the student starts on his first quick 'run' through the questions by filling in all the answers he knows to be correct. On this first 'run' he should also mark (on the paper) the questions where he is fully acquainted with the material but is unsure of the correct response. On the second 'run' all his attention can now be given to this group of questions, in which he should be able to make an informed guess. Experience has shown that his chances of being correct in this situation are above average. He should, as one examiner expresses it, 'play his hunches'. The questions which he does not understand are probably best left unanswered as at best he can only hope for a 50 per cent chance of a correct response on a random basis in the true/false situation, and only a 25 per cent chance of a correct response in a four-item multiple choice question. In multiple choice questions the marking is usually positive, a mark being given for a correct answer and none for an incorrect one. In multiple response questions (as in this text) a mark is given for each correct response, whether this be true or false, and usually a mark is subtracted for each incorrect response. Most examination systems have now abolished the use of a correction factor for guessing as this was found to have little effect on the ranking of the candidates, it has also been realised that informed guessing is in itself a useful discrimination.

Lack of time is not usually a problem in medical objective testing. Since these tests are of the 'power' rather than the 'speed' variety, i.e. knowledge rather than ability against the clock is being tested. Excessive time may be a disadvantage to the candidate as repeated reassessment of the answers may distract from the correct response rather than produce improvement. In the multiple choice situation it has been found that one minute is usually necessary per question although more time is required to answer a question containing a number of distractors.

Transcribing 300 items from a question paper to an answer sheet (i.e. 60 questions each with 5 options) takes a minimum of 10 minutes and the habit of leaving such transcriptions to the end of an examination is best avoided since, if rushed, it may introduce unnecessary inaccuracies.

Etymological Hazards

The rarity of absolutes in medicine means that a large variety of adjectives and adverbs are commonly used in its description. These increase the difficulty of both setting and answering multiple choice questions. Although one can question the desirability of assessing knowledge which is dependent on the 'strength of an adjective', these adjectives do form the language of present day medical practice. This factor is borne out by their frequent use in the questions and answers of the present text. Nevertheless, the examiner must avoid ambiguity and in addition his questions must not contain clues to the correct answer. Such terms as 'invariable', 'always', 'must', 'all', 'only', and 'never' should be avoided since they imply absolutes and are therefore likely to be wrong.

The terms 'may' and 'can' also give rise to ambiguity. In medicine almost anything 'may occur' and statements using this phrase are unlikely to be completely wrong. If these terms are used and the student is able to answer that the question 'certainly may' or 'certainly may not', he has little chance of being wrong. The term 'sometimes' comes into the same category.

The adjectives and adverbs 'common', 'usual', 'frequent' (commonly, usually, frequently), 'likely' and 'often' are an integral part of everyday medical language but their use in the multiple choice question may also lead to ambiguity. Their meanings are very similar yet their values depend largely on the context of the question. Expressed as incidences they may well range from 30 to 70 per cent. They may be considerably modified by the addition of 'quite', 'most', 'very' and 'extremely'. The examiner must be particularly careful of his choice of these terms. The 'majority' implies more than 50 per cent, whereas the 'vast majority' implies nearly 100 per cent.

The term 'typical' is a useful one for multiple choice questions. Its meaning implies 'that which is found in clinical practice'. 'Characteristic' implies a time honoured diagnostic feature and 'recognised' an accepted text book feature. Less explicit, and therefore less desirable, terminology includes 'most authorities agree', 'generally assumed', 'probable', 'thought to be', 'all reports indicate' and 'has recently been reported'. Further vague terminology used in medical practice yet best avoided in the multiple choice situation include 'associated with', 'accompanied by', 'related to', 'linked with' and 'lend support to'.

On the negative side, 'uncommon', 'unusual', 'infrequent' (uncommonly, unusually, infrequently), 'unlikely' and 'rare' are all terms commonly used yet their use in the multiple choice situation must not give rise to ambiguity. As with their positive equivalents they are markedly influenced by the addition of such terms as 'most' and 'very'. The term 'significant' is best kept for its statistical use and the terms 'increased' and 'more' should be restricted to direct comparative situations.

The terms 'demand' and 'should' indicate the examiner's personal opinion and, although their inclusion is questionable, the student is still required to indicate whether he thinks the opinion is valid.

In conclusion, words used in multiple choice questions, although giving rise to apparent ambiguity, remain those in common use in medical practice; both the examiner and the student must be fully conversant with their meanings and disadvantages in order to avoid any confusion. It is hoped that the questions which follow will also help in this regard.

Contents

How to use this book

The text, consisting of questions and answers ('true or false'), is arranged throughout in such a way that all questions appear on left-hand pages and all answers on right-hand pages.

In use the student may conveniently cover the right-hand page with a blank sheet on which to jot down his answers for comparison.

I Fluid and Electrolyte Balance

1 The normal adult value for:

a Urine output is 1.5 litre/day.   (   )
b Insensible water loss is 200 ml/day.   (   )

c Potassium requirement is 150 mEq (150 mmol)/day.   (   )

d Protein requirement is 70 g/day.   (   )

2 In a healthy 70 kg male the:

a Total body water measures approximately 40 litres.   (   )

b Extracellular fluid volume measures approximately 8 litres.   (   )

c Plasma volume measures approximately 3.5 litres.   (   )
d 'Third space' fluid measures approximately 1 litre.   (   )

3 The pH of the extracellular fluid:

a Is maintained in health between 7.4 and 7.6.   (   )
b Is maintained entirely by the buffering system of the intra-   (   )
  and extra-cellular fluids.

c Is increased in hypovolaemic shock.   (   )
d Decreases abruptly after a cardiac arrest.   (   )

4 A low serum sodium level:

a Is commonly present in the early postoperative period.   (   )

b May cause stupor and fits.   (   )
c Should be treated with isotonic saline infusions.   (   )
d Is associated with an impaired ability to excrete water.   (   )

a   T— In a temperate climate.

b   F— Insensible loss via skin and lungs ranges from 700 to 1000 ml/day and will be increased during fever and high ambient temperatures.

c   F— Potassium requirements of the healthy adult are 40 to 60 mEq (40 to 60 mmol)/day. There are excessive losses during starvation, hypercatabolic states, intestinal obstruction and diarrhoea.

d   T— This is increased in hypercatabolic states such as burns and severe sepsis.

a   T— The average values are 62 per cent of total body weight in males and 52 per cent in females.

b   F— The extracellular fluid volume measures about 22 per cent of the body weight, i.e. approximately 15 litres. This includes plasma volume, lymph and interstitial fluid.

c   T— The whole blood volume being approximately 5 litres.

d   T— This is the fluid normally in the pleural and peritoneal cavities and the cerebrospinal fluid together with the secretions in the alimentary tract. This component enlarges considerably at the expense of the extracellular fluid volume in peritonitis, intestinal obstruction and with any large inflammatory area.

a   F— In the healthy individual the pH is maintained between 7.35 and 7.42

b   F   by the buffering capacity of the bicarbonate/carbonic acid system, the phosphate buffer system and the buffering properties of the serum proteins and haemoglobin. Additional regulation is by the lungs and kidneys.

c   F— Shock is always associated with a metabolic acidosis.

d   T— The absence of tissue perfusion results in a rapid fall in the pH of the extracellular fluid.

a   T— Increased antidiuretic hormone production occurs resulting in increased water retention.

b   T— This complication may be confused with a cerebrovascular accident.

c   F— 3 per cent (hypertonic) saline should be administered in order to

d   T   produce a diuresis and overcome the inability of the kidney to excrete water in hyponatraemia.

5 **The sodium ion:**

a   Is the principal regulator of the intracellular volume.   (   )

b   Is the major ionic component of the extracellular fluid   (   )
volume.

c   Is present in greater concentration in intracellular fluid   (   )
than extracellular fluid.

d   Is excreted in larger amounts than normal in the early   (   )
postoperative period.

6 **Potassium deficiency should be suspected:**

a   In cases of paralytic ileus.   (   )

b   When the patient's reflexes are exaggerated.   (   )

c   If there is an increase in height and peaking of the T waves   (   )
of an ECG.

d   In alkalotic states.   (   )

7 **Potassium deficiency:**

a   Can be effectively monitored by the serum potassium   (   )
levels.

b   May render digitalis therapy more dangerous.   (   )

c   Should be treated with an infusion of normal saline with   (   )
potassium supplements.

d   Is not usually present in intestinal obstruction.   (   )

8 **The effects of a major extracellular fluid deficiency:**

a   Include a decreased skin turgor.   (   )

b   Include hypotension.   (   )

c   Include excessive salivation.   (   )

d   May be corrected by an infusion of isotonic saline.   (   )

a T— Because of the low intracellular concentration of sodium, ionic
b T   movement of the ion into or out of the extracellular fluid is
       accompanied by an immediate movement of fluid into or out of
       the intracellular space.
c F— Sodium is almost exclusively an extracellular ion.

d F— There is an initial postoperative retention of sodium.

a T— Potassium deficiency may be both a cause and an effect of paralytic
       ileus. A diminished intracellular potassium results in atony of both
       visceral and skeletal muscle.
b F— The reflexes are decreased.
c F— The myocardium is also subject to muscle atony and an ECG shows a
       prolongation of the Q–T interval, depression of the ST segment and
       eventual inversion of the T wave.
d T— When there is excessive chloride loss, potassium excretion rises as the
       kidney attempts to conserve hydrogen ions.

a F— The major store of potassium is intracellular and the serum levels may
       be normal in the presence of a large intracellular deficit.
b T— Potassium deficiency enhances the effect of digitalis and dysrhythmias
       are prone to occur.
c T— The infusion should not contain more than 40 mEq (40 mmol) of
       potassium/litre and should usually not be administered at more than
       15 mEq (15 mmol) potassium/hour.
d F— A deficient intake and excessive losses of potassium into the bowel
       lumen often lead to potassium deficiency in this condition.

a T— These are due to the resultant hypovolaemia.
b T
c F— The mucous membranes are drier than normal.
d T— This solution and other isotonic electrolyte-containing fluids such as
       Ringer's lactate are the most effective agents for restoring extracellular
       fluid.

9   **Extracellular fluid losses are often extensive in:**
a   Intestinal obstruction.   (   )
b   Peritonitis.   (   )
c   Pancreatitis.   (   )
d   Hepatic coma.   (   )

10   **Excessive vomiting or loss of gastric secretion by
        nasogastric suction:**
a   Produces a metabolic alkalosis.   (   )
b   Results in a low serum potassium.   (   )
c   May produce renal failure.   (   )
d   Should be treated with isotonic saline infusions.   (   )

11   **Increases in the extracellular fluid volume can be accurately assessed
        and fluid overloading avoided by:**
a   Serum electrolyte determinations.   (   )

b   The measurement of the central venous pressure (CVP).   (   )

c   The measurement of hourly urine volumes.   (   )
d   Serial body weighing.   (   )

12   **Anuria in the postoperative period:**
a   Is defined as the production of less than 500 ml of urine/day. (   )

b   Should be treated with an initial 'waterload', i.e. a 4 litre   (   )
    fluid infusion.
c   Is associated with hypernatraemia and dehydration.   (   )

d   Is usually treated by renal dialysis.   (   )

a   T– In all these conditions there may be extensive internal translocations
b   T   of fluid from the extracellular compartment to the 'third space' (see Q.2).
c   T
d   F– In liver failure the extracellular fluid volume is usually increased.

a   T– There is an excessive loss of hydrogen and chloride ions producing an
b   T   alkalosis. As the loss of chloride continues the kidney is unable to
c   T   reabsorb the tubular sodium and substitutes potassium in the tubular
d   T   urine. Thus potassium excretion rises and serum potassium falls. The
associated loss of fluid often gives rise to uraemia. These metabolic
upsets usually respond to infusions of isotonic saline but occasionally
potassium needs to be added.

a   F– Normal values are often found in patients with severe abnormalities of
extracellular fluid volume.
b   F– In chronic hypervolaemia the CVP may not be raised as the bulk of
the fluid will lie in the interstitial space rather than in the plasma.
c   F– There is often some associated renal failure.
d   T– This investigation will reveal extracellular fluid increases prior to the
development of pulmonary and sacral oedema. It is particularly useful
in the management of chronic hepatic, renal and cardiac problems. In
the acutely fluid depleted patient, however, all these factors (a to d)
are helpful in assessing fluid requirements.

a   F– This is the definition of oliguria. Anuria is defined as the production of
less than 100 ml/day.
b   F– In the absence of hypovolaemia immediate fluid restriction should be
instituted.
c   F– There is almost always overhydration, relative haemodilution and a low
serum sodium level.
d   F– Most patients should have precise fluid therapy based on a policy of
replacing only insensible and urinary losses. Cases of refractory renal
tubular necrosis may be considered for short term dialysis.

13   The anuric patient:

a   Should have a fluid intake of 1 to 1.5 litres per day.   (   )

b   Should have no potassium administered.   (   )

c   Is at risk from metabolic alkalosis.   (   )

d   Should be on continuous urinary catheter drainage.   (   )

14   Acute post traumatic renal failure:

a   May be due to hypovolaemia and poor tissue perfusion.   (   )

b   Is particularly associated with crush injuries.   (   )

c   May be due to kidney damage following tubular   (   )
obstruction.

d   Should initially be treated by fluid restriction.   (   )

15   Intravenous parenteral feeding:

a   Should deliver at least 2500 calories/day to an adult.   (   )

b   Should deliver at least 10 g of nitrogen (i.e. 66 g of protein)/   (   )
day to an adult.

c   Can be effectively achieved with isotonic solutions.   (   )

d   Is without complications with present day solutions and   (   )
methods of administration.

a F— Only insensible losses should be replaced. These will range from 400 to 700 ml/day.
b T— A rising serum potassium is one of the more serious effects of anuria. When it rises above 6 mEq (6mmol)/l exchange resins should be administered orally or rectally and dialysis considered.
c F— Metabolic acidosis is almost always present and is due to the accumulation of sulphates and phosphates.
d F— Catheterisation should be avoided unless specific surgical indications are present. This will reduce the risk of urinary infection.

a T— Any prolonged decrease in extracellular fluid volume and tissue
b T perfusion will result in renal dysfunction. This may also be due to
c T tubular obstruction by blood pigments following crush injuries, mismatched transfusions or burns.
d F— It is desirable to give a provocative test, such as 1 litre of dextrose intravenously in 90 minutes where hypovolaemia is suspected. Similarly, the initial treatment of tubular necrosis should include a fluid load and diuretics. Only when these methods fail should fluids be restricted.

a T— The ideal solution has not yet been found but the proteins should be in
b T the form of amino acids and the calorie source as carbohydrate and, to a lesser extent, alcohol. Emulsified fat may also be used.
c F— The tolerable limit for water intake in a sick patient is of the order of 3 litres; thus the solutions used, in order to supply the requisite amount of calories and amino acids must be hypertonic.
d F— Thrombophlebitis and septicaemia are frequent complications, diminished to some extent by the use of large veins and the use of a scrupulous sterile technique when setting up the infusion. Hyperosmolar coma is occasionally seen.

16 **Tube feeding of a complete low bulk diet:**
a   Results in constipation. ( )

b   Often results in uraemia and dehydration. ( )

c   Carries the risk of gastric reflux and pulmonary ( )
    complications.
d   Is ineffective as a long term method of nutrition. ( )

II Shock and Blood Transfusion

17 **'Shock' can be most comprehensively defined as:**
a   A sudden large volume blood loss. ( )

b   A diminished effective circulating fluid volume. ( )
c   A hypotensive state with peripheral vasoconstriction. ( )
d   An unexpected psychological insult. ( )

18 **In all forms of shock there is:**
a   An impairment of cellular oxygenation. ( )
b   A decreased cardiac output. ( )
c   A diminished effective circulating fluid volume. ( )
d   A low central venous pressure (CVP). ( )

19 **The pulmonary insufficiency, frequently seen in shock,
      may be caused by:**
a   An increased pulmonary capillary permeability. ( )
b   Cardiac failure. ( )
c   Fluid overload. ( )

d   A reduced minute volume. ( )

a   F–   Diarrhoea is common with hyperosmolar diets. It should be treated by reducing the rate of administration.

b   T–   The feeds are often hyperosmolar and excessive fluid losses in the faeces and urine may produce prerenal uraemia and dehydration.

c   T–   Rapid administration of fluid may be accompanied by regurgitation and aspiration of gastric contents.

d   F–   With due precautions to avoid the above complications, this is a satisfactory method for long term nutrition.

a   F–   This definition is incomplete. It does not include shock due to plasma or water loss, cardiogenic causes or shock which accompanies generalised septicaemia.

b   T–   This is the most comprehensive definition.

c   F–   Early bacteraemic shock is often characterised by warm extremities.

d   F–   This lay use of the term is irrelevant in the clinical situation.

a   T–   This is present in all forms of shock.

b   F–   The cardiac output is raised in early septicaemic shock.

c   T–   This is a comprehensive definition of the syndrome.

d   F–   In cases of cardiogenic shock the CVP is usually elevated.

a   T–   No single cause of the shock lung has been identified. All these factors

b   T   together with fat embolism, oxygen toxicity and multiple microemboli

c   T   in the pulmonary vessels may play a part. The frequent finding of pulmonary oedema in the absence of a raised central venous pressure or a decreased serum albumin, suggests that increased capillary permeability is the major cause. In cardiogenic shock and late hypovolaemia, cardiac failure plays a part. Fluid overload may occur and produce pulmonary oedema without right heart failure.

d   F–   The patient is usually hyperventilating and the minute volume is increased.

20 **Important and urgent measures in the diagnosis and treatment of shock are:**
a Warming the patient. ( )

b Measurement of the central venous pressure. ( )
c Noting the response of the central venous pressure to a ( )
rapid infusion of 200 to 500 ml of fluid.
d Urinary catheterisation. ( )

21 **The metabolic acidosis of shock can be effectively treated by:**
a Warming the patient. ( )
b Administering sodium bicarbonate. ( )
c Artifical ventilation. ( )
d Restoring normal tissue perfusion. ( )

22 **In hypovolaemic shock:**
a The central venous pressure is low. ( )
b The difference in arteriovenous oxygen tension is ( )
unaffected.
c The extremities are pale, cold and sweating. ( )
d Urine output is unaffected. ( )

23 **Hypovolaemic shock may result from:**
a A 25 per cent third degree burn. ( )

b Generalised peritonitis. ( )

c Massive pulmonary embolism. ( )

d Intestinal obstruction. ( )

a F— Though the skin vessels are usually contracted and the extremities cold this should be recognised as an effect rather than the cause of shock. Effective treatment will restore normal circulation.

b T— It is important to ensure that the right atrial filling pressure is sufficient

c T to produce a normal cardiac output. The response of the central venous pressure to a rapid fluid infusion is often necessary to

d T distinguish cardiogenic from other forms of shock and normally the hourly urine volume will drop below 50 ml/hour when inadequate tissue perfusion is present.

a F— The basic cause of the acidosis is poor tissue perfusion and unless this is

b T corrected there can be no permanent improvement. Bicarbonate is

c F only necessary in cases of severe acidosis when a pH of below 7.1 may

d T lead to serious cardiac arrhythmias.

a T— This is due to the low circulating fluid volume.

b F— The associated decreased cardiac output leads to an increased arteriovenous difference in oxygen tension.

c T— This is due to reflex sympathetic stimulae.

d F— The hourly urine volume falls because of decreased renal perfusion. Treatment should aim to maintain urine outflow at about 50 ml/hr.

a T— This is due to excessive sequestration of fluid in the burned area and to serum losses.

b T— This is due to fluid sequestration in the inflamed peritoneum and adynamic bowel.

c F— There is no change in the extracellular volume in this condition although cardiogenic shock frequently follows the reduced cardiac output.

d T— Hypovolaemia results from excessive fluid loss due to fluid sequestration in the distended bowel.

24   Appropriate *immediate* intravenous infusions in all
      cases of non-cardiogenic shock are:
a   Whole blood.   (   )
b   Ringer's lactate.   (   )
c   Normal saline.   (   )

d   Low molecular weight dextran.   (   )

25   Oliguria occuring in a shocked patient after the central
      venous pressure and blood pressure have been corrected
      to normal may require:
a   Frusemide 40 mg intravenously.   (   )
b   Mannitol 20 g in 200 ml 5 per cent dextrose.   (   )

c   An increased fluid intake.   (   )
d   Potassium supplements.   (   )

26   The following vasoactive drugs may be used intravenously
      with benefit in the shocked patient:
a   Adrenaline.   (   )
b   Noradrenaline.   (   )

c   Isoprenaline.   (   )

d   Phenoxybenzamine.   (   )

27   Septic shock:
a   Is only caused by gram-negative organisms.   (   )

b   Carries a favourable prognosis.   (   )
c   Produces a cellular defect that inhibits oxygen utilisation. (   )
d   Is particularly associated with infective complications of   (   )
      the gastrointestinal and genito-urinary systems.

a   F— This should be restricted to cases of blood loss.
b   T— Both of these isotonic fluids satisfactorily expand the plasma volume.
c   T   The serum electrolytes should be estimated as soon as possible to assess the long term requirements. The haematocrit should be checked to assess the need for blood.
d   T— Though this fluid has few advantages over Ringer's lactate or saline and can produce spontaneous bleeding and crossmatching problems.

a   T— Both these diuretics can be used. If there is no diuresis after 30
b   T   minutes, frusemide may then be given again in a dose of up to 600 mg. If there is still no effect serious renal damage should be suspected and a regime of fluid restriction instituted.
c   F— This may result in fluid overload.
d   F— Serum potassium levels rise in renal failure and may be lethal.

a   F— Both these drugs increase peripheral resistance and decrease cardiac
b   F   output. Their use in shock is detrimental. Intracardiac adrenaline may be used in the treatment of ventricular asystole.
c   T— In some forms of cardiogenic shock (where bradycardia is present) and in advanced hypovolaemic shock with associated heart failure this drug may be helpful.
d   T— This vasodilator may increase cardiac output. It should only be given to patients who are not hypovolaemic and whose CVP is being monitored.

a   F— Although the commonest organisms are gram-negative, gram-positive organisms and fungi may also cause septic shock.
b   F— The mortality usually exceeds 30 per cent.
c   T— This may precede the haemodynamic changes.
d   T— This incidence is further increased by instrumental or surgical manipulation of the infected region.

28 **Septic shock is particularly associated with:**
 a Thoracic surgical patients. ( )
 b Hypovolaemia. ( )
 c Indwelling urinary or intravenous catheters. ( )
 d Gram-negative bacteraemia. ( )

29 **Early septic shock is commonly associated with:**
 a A high central venous pressure. ( )
 b A high cardiac output. ( )
 c A low blood pressure. ( )
 d Cold sweaty extremities. ( )

30 **The presence of spontaneous haemorrhage in septic shock suggests:**
 a Hypovolaemia. ( )
 b Liver failure. ( )
 c Excessive fibrinolysis. ( )
 d Disseminated intravascular coagulation (DIC). ( )

31 **Septic shock is associated with a hypodynamic cardiovascular state:**
 a If preceded by existing hypovolaemia. ( )
 b In generalised peritonitis. ( )

 c When there is a gram-positive bacteraemia. ( )

 d In elderly patients. ( )

a	F—	Both medical and surgical patients are at risk, particularly those with
b	T	hypovolaemia, septic foci and indwelling intravenous cannulae or
c	T	urinary catheters. 30 per cent of patients with a gram-negative
d	T	bacteraemia develop septic shock and this is commoner in patients

with widespread neoplasia and in patients over the age of 50.

a	T—	Hyperdynamic or 'warm' shock is a frequent early pattern in septic
b	T	shock. This is associated with hyperventilation and a low blood pressure.
c	T	The extremities are warm and dry due to vasodilatation and a higher
d	F	than normal cardiac output.

a	F—	Not associated.
b	F—	Not associated.
c	T—	Endotoxin may accelerate the clotting process to produce DIC which
d	T	in its turn can produce spontaneous haemorrhages, pulmonary oedema

and pancreatitis. Excessive fibrinolysis may be associated with DIC, but
may occur independently. Treatment of DIC may require fresh blood
transfusions and possibly heparinisation.

a	T—	In all cases where sepsis complicates a process producing a loss of
b	T	extracellular fluid volume such as peritonitis, gangrenous bowel and

intestinal obstruction, the hypodynamic pattern of shock is seen with a
low central venous pressure, low cardiac output and cold sweaty
extremities.

c	F—	This form of septic shock characteristically produces a hyperdynamic
		state.
d	T—	These patients are particularly prone to septic shock.

32   **The diminished oxygen consumption in patients with septic shock is due to:**

a   Failure of oxygen transport in the lungs.   (   )

b   Diminished blood flow in the periphery.   (   )

c   Arteriovenous shunting in the periphery.   (   )

d   Diminished oxygen utilisation by the cells.   (   )

33   **The mortality from septic shock can be effectively reduced by:**

a   Surgical drainage of abscesses.   (   )
b   The administration of appropriate antibiotics.   (   )
c   The restoration of a normal cardiovascular state.   (   )

d   Positive pressure respiration via a tracheostomy.   (   )

34   **In cardiogenic shock:**

a   The central venous pressure is low.   (   )
b   The difference in the arteriovenous oxygen tension is increased.   (   )
c   The haematocrit is raised.   (   )

d   The blood pressure is unaffected.   (   )

35   **Prospective blood donors:**

a   Should be asked about previous attacks of jaundice.   (   )

b   Should have serological tests for syphilis.   (   )

c   May transmit glandular fever to a recipient.   (   )
d   May transmit malaria to a recipient.   (   )

a T— The pulmonary oedema associated with septic shock impairs oxygen uptake.
b F— Even in hyperdynamic states, where peripheral blood flow is increased, there is a deficient oxygen uptake due to impaired cellular functions.
c F— Xenon clearance studies have not shown any peripheral arteriovenous shunting in these patients.
d T— Vital cell functions are impaired with a resultant inability to utilise oxygen.

a T— Patients have a better prognosis after drainage.
b T— The mortality rate is halved when effective antibiotics are used.
c T— This may require blood or saline infusions and possibly the administration of isoprenaline and digitalis.
d T— Mechanical ventilation should not be restricted to those patients with specific respiratory indications.

a F— There is usually an increased central venous pressure.
b T— This is due to inadequate tissue perfusion.

c F— The haematocrit is unchanged whereas in hypovolaemic shock not due to blood loss it is raised.
d F— The inadequate cardiac output always produces a fall in blood pressure.

a T— Donors who have had serum or infective hepatitis may remain infective for up to 3 years.
b T— Spirochaetes are transmissible (they will survive for 4 days in stored blood). Gonorrhoea is not transmissible.
c T— This infection is transmissible.
d T— In some countries malarial donors are not accepted although the serum alone may be used without risk of transmission.

36 **A blood transfusion reaction:**
a May be due to incompatibility of the recipient serum and donor cells. ( )
b Is manifest by thrombophlebitis of the infusion site. ( )

c Occurs within the first 30 minutes of transfusion. ( )

d May produce renal damage. ( )

37 **Pyrexial reactions to blood transfusions:**
a Have increased since the introduction of sterile disposable infusion sets. ( )
b May be caused by allergic reactions. ( )
c May be caused by contaminated blood. ( )

d May be a response to a large transfusion of cooled blood. ( )

38 **Massive blood transfusions may be complicated by:**
a Hyperkalaemia. ( )

b Hypercalcaemia. ( )

c Hepatic coma. ( )

d Leucopenia ( )

III Burns

39 **When determining the depth of a burn:**
a A knowledge of the type of injury is important. ( )

b The presence of blisters is of no clinical significance. ( )
c Impairment of sensibility of the burned area should be tested. ( )
d The presence of severe pain denotes a full thickness skin loss. ( )

a T— Mismatching produces agglutination of the donor cells.

b F— The signs include fever, chills, breathlessness and pain in the flanks and chest. These may be followed by hypotension, haemorrhagic phenoma and haemoglobinuria.

c T— This period should be closely observed when a blood transfusion is commenced.

d T— This is the result of haemoglobinuria, hypotension and acidosis. It should be treated by immediately stopping the transfusion, invoking a diuresis and restoring the patient's blood pressure.

a F— Pyrogen reactions have decreased since the introduction of disposable infusion sets.

b T— This is due to allergens in the donor blood.

c T— Gram-negative endotoxins are the commonest cause and bacteria may multiply in warm blood. Blood should therefore be stored at 4°C until it is required.

d F— This produces a fall in body temperature.

a T— In 3-week-old blood the plasma potassium rises to 30 to 40 mEq (30 to 40 mmol)/litre.

b F— Hypocalcaemia may occur and this is accentuated if citrate is used as the anticoagulant. It should be treated by the administration of calcium chloride.

c T— This may occur in cirrhotic patients, possibly due to a high ammonia concentration.

d F— There is no change in the white cell count.

a T— Contact with hot liquids usually causes partial thickness loss, whereas flames commonly give rise to full thickness losses.

b F— Blisters do not occur in full thickness loss.

c T— Full thickness burns have a reduced pain sensibility.

d F— Nerve endings in the area of a full thickness burn are usually destroyed.

true or false

40 **Estimation of the area of a burn:**
a Is of very little clinical significance. ( )

b Provides important prognostic information. ( )
c Is an important factor in the estimation of the fluid ( )
required.

d Can be based on a formula which states that the adult ( )
trunk is 36 per cent of the whole body surface area.

41 **Patients with major burns:**
a Are in a negative nitrogen balance. ( )

b Have normal calorie requirements. ( )

c Do not generally become anaemic. ( )

d Are resistant to septicaemia. ( )

42 **The catabolic response to trauma and infection is characterised by:**
a An increase in lean body mass. ( )
b A positive nitrogen balance. ( )
c Gluconeogenesis. ( )
d A falling haemoglobin level. ( )

43 **The catabolic response to trauma:**
a Is related to the severity of the trauma. ( )

b Is accompanied by increased urinary losses of ( )
potassium and nitrogen.
c Can be prevented by parenteral nutrition. ( )

d Does not occur in the adrenalectomised patient. ( )

a   F— The form of therapy and the fluid requirements of the patient are determined by the area of the burn.
b   T— The prognosis after a burn injury is related to the extent of the burn.
c   T— This is an important guide, although no formula for fluid therapy in burns can be precise. It is also important to carefully monitor indices of tissue perfusion and cardiovascular status, such as hourly urine volume and central venous pressure measurements.
d   T— The 'Rule of Nines' wherein the head and upper limbs each measure 9 per cent and the lower limbs 18 per cent each is widely used as a rough guide in estimating the area of a burn.

a   T— Even if the greatly increased needs of 150 to 200 g protein/day are met the negative nitrogen balance will persist until the wound is healed.
b   F— Calorie requirements may be at least twice normal due to increased energy losses such as through increased evaporative water loss and fever. Parenteral nutrition is thus frequently necessary.
c   F— There is blood destruction and sequestration in the early days of a burn. These factors together with infection and septicaemia give rise to anaemia.
d   F— They have an increased subsceptibility to infection and have many more potential sources of infection than a healthy patient.

a   F— A breakdown of tissue protein provides substrates for gluconeogenesis.
b   F   There is thus a loss of most body tissue proteins, this being reflected
c   T   by a decrease of the lean body mass and a negative nitrogen balance.
d   F— Haemoglobin synthesis is usually unaffected in the catabolic phase.

a   T— Whereas a patient with a fractured femur will lose approximately 11 g of nitrogen (70 g of protein)/day, a major burn may lose 40 g of nitrogen/day.
b   T— Following protein catabolism and gluconeogenesis.

c   F— Parenterally administered amino acids when suitably admixed with a source of calories minimise but do not abolish the catabolic response.
d   F— There is no known dependance on the endocrine system.

44   **Scalds:**

a   Are more frequent in children.   (   )

b   Commonly cause full thickness skin loss.   (   )

c   Should be skin grafted within 48 hours of the injury.   (   )

d   Need routine antibiotic treatment.   (   )

45   **The dressing of a small burn should be:**

a   Occlusive.   (   )

b   Non-absorbtive.   (   )

c   Non-compressive.   (   )

d   Changed daily as a routine.   (   )

46   **A partial thickness burn:**

a   May heal without grafting.   (   )

b   May deteriorate into full thickness skin loss.   (   )

c   Rarely causes severe physiological derangement of the patient.   (   )

d   Heals within 7 days in the absence of infection.   (   )

47   **Fluid losses in a major burn:**

a   Are maximal between 12 and 24 hours after the injury.   (   )

b   Are related to the age of the patient.   (   )

c   Are related to the weight of the patient.   (   )

d   Are related to the area burnt.   (   )

a T— This is especially so in children under 3 years of age.
b F— Hot or boiling water usually produces partial skin loss.
c F— Local cleansing and the application of a non-adherent sterile dressing
d F   are all that is usually required. Healing generally takes place
       uneventfully without the need for grafting or antibiotic therapy.

a T— The aim of the dressing is to prevent bacterial invasion and to provide
b F   firm compression and support. If these criteria are met, it need only
c F   be changed every 4 or 5 days. The infected burn will require
d F   dressing daily or more frequently.

a T— Epithelial regeneration will spread from the epithelial remnants in the
       hair follicles and deeper layers of the epidermis.
b T— Infection may convert it into a full thickness skin loss by destroying
       the remaining dermal elements.
c F— In a deep partial thickness burn there is a considerable inflammatory
       response even though some epidermal elements may have escaped
       injury. If the burn is of more than 15 to 20 per cent of the body
       surface, hypovolaemia may develop.
d F— The deeper partial thickness burns may require 3 or 4 weeks before
       epithelial regeneration is complete.

a F— Are maximal in the first 8 hours after burning.
b F— There is no known relationship to age but there is a direct relationship to
c T   body weight, the area burnt and the depth of the burn. Many guides to
d T   fluid therapy in the burned patient take account of these factors, e.g:
           First 24 hours:
           (i) electrolyte solution 1.5 ml/kg/per cent body surface burn
           (ii) colloid solution 0.5 ml/kg/per cent body surface burn.
       Plus metabolic requirements (approximately 2000 ml in an adult).
       Half the above fluid is given intravenously in the first 8 hours and one
       quarter in each of the successive 8 hours.

48   **The increased fluid requirements of a patient with a full thickness burn are due to:**

a   Increased evaporative water loss.   (   )

b   Sequestration of fluid in the injured tissues.   (   )

c   Serum exuding from the burned area.   (   )

d   Destruction of blood in the skin vessels.   (   )

49   **48 hours after a major burn and with satisfactory fluid therapy a patient:**

a   Has very few abnormal fluid losses.   (   )

b   May need a blood transfusion.   (   )

c   Is often hypernatraemic.   (   )

d   Usually needs skin grafting.   (   )

50   **Major burns are sometimes complicated by:**

a   Acute gastric and duodenal ulcers.   (   )

b   Paralytic ileus.   (   )

c   Cerebral oedema.   (   )

d   Mesenteric thrombosis.   (   )

51   **In a burned patient, associated pulmonary injury:**

a   Should be suspected in head and neck burns.   (   )

b   Should be suspected when the nasal hairs are burnt.   (   )

c   Does not appear clinically in the first 24 hours.   (   )

d   May be avoided by the prophylactic use of antibiotics. (   )

a T— Evaporative water loss from a full thickness burn is more than 10 times
b T   that of intact skin. Two and a half litres of water may be lost per day
c T   from a 40 per cent burn. There is a local (and to a lesser extent, a
       general) increase in capillary permeability so that protein-rich fluid
       gains the interstitial space from the blood. Large amounts of fluid are
       sequestrated in the inflammation which surrounds the burn injury.
       Relatively little serum is lost from a full thickness burn.
d F— Although there is some destruction of red cells and a diminution in the
       red cell mass this is not an important factor in accounting for the
       increased fluid requirements.

a F— Insensible evaporative water loss is still excessive—up to 3 litres/day in
       the adult with extensive burns.
b T— Destruction of red cells, trapping of blood in thrombosed capillaries
       and increased phagocytosis of red cells may produce anaemia at this
       time.
c T— This is mainly due to increased insensible losses of water.
d F— Surgical debridement of a major burn at this time is very traumatic and
       is rarely indicated. Skin grafting is sometimes undertaken after 7 days
       but there is a need for great care in limiting the blood loss.

a T— The ulcers are known as Curling's ulcers. They are frequently multiple
       in the stomach and most common in extensive burns.
b T— This often lasts 48 to 72 hours.
c T— This is maximal 48 to 72 hours after the injury when the risk of
       hyponatraemia due to over-transfusion with intravenous fluids is
       greatest.
d F— There is no recognised relationship.

a T— The additional sign of pharyngeal inflammation may be present and
b T   should be looked for.
c F— The effects of burn injury to the lungs are often immediate.
d F— Antibiotics do not prevent the injury but may prevent secondary
       infection.

52   Secondary infection of burns:

a   Is less common in partial than in full thickness skin loss.   (   )

b   Is relatively more common in burns of more than 20 per   (   )
      cent body area.

c   Is avoided by leaving the burn eschar intact.   (   )

d   Is avoided by the immediate application of a sterile   (   )
      occlusive dressing.

53   The early management of a burn wound may include:

a   Early excision.   (   )

b   Occlusive dressings.   (   )

c   Exposure treatment.   (   )

d   Dressings with local antibiotics.   (   )

54   Skin grafting of a burn wound:

a   Should usually be with full thickness skin grafts.   (   )

b   Is more likely to be successful if undertaken in the first   (   )
      week after injury.

c   Will be unsuccessful unless the wound surface is sterile.   (   )

d   Minimises scar contracture.   (   )

55   The prognosis of a burned patient is:

a   Related to the patient's age.   (   )

b   Related to the area burnt.   (   )

c   Generally better below the age of 10 years.   (   )

d   Very poor in the patient with burns of over 40 per cent   (   )
      surface area.

a   **T—** The protective function of the skin against invasive infection by
b   **F**   environmental organisms is lost when a full thickness burn is present.
To a large extent this protective function is retained in a partial
thickness burn. Small burns are as readily infected as large burns.
c   **F—** The dry dead burn eschar is permeable and is an entry site for invasive
infection.
d   **F—** Viable bacteria may remain in the follicles deep to the burned surface
and subsequently multiply to infect the area.

a   **T—** All these treatments are acceptable depending on the type of burn.
b   **T**   Minor partial thickness burns may warrant outpatient
c   **T**   management with occlusive dressings and small full thickness
d   **T**   burns early excision. In major burns fluid therapy has priority
and the burn is treated as the circumstances dictate.

a   **F—** With the exception of very small burns of the eyelids or the delayed
treatment of contractures (when full thickness pedicle grafts may be
used), split thickness skin grafts are used.
b   **F—** Grafting is less successful before granulation tissue is present.
However homo- or hetero-graft skin may be used as a very effective
burn dressing in the early stages of repair.
c   **F—** Although beta-haemolytic streptococci are inimical to skin grafts,
moderate infections of the wound with other organisms are not a
contra-indication to skin grafting.
d   **T—** For this reason burns around joints should receive early attention.

a   **T—** After middle age the prognosis worsens with advancing years.
b   **T—** There is a direct relationship; the larger the burn the worse the
prognosis.
c   **F—** Young children have a higher mortality rate than adults in burns of
equivalent size.
d   **F—** 40 per cent survival rates have been recorded in series of patients
with 60 per cent burns and occasional survivors are reported in
patients with more than 70 per cent burns.

IV Wound Healing, Surgical Infection and Postoperative Complications

56 A clean incised skin wound:

a Undergoes an inflammatory phase during the processes of repair. ( )

b Commences epithelialization after 7 to 10 days. ( )

c Regains the full strength of normal skin within 10 days. ( )

d Regains its strength as the result of fibroblast activity. ( )

57 Wound healing:

a Is impaired in anaemic patients. ( )

b Is impaired by haematoma formation. ( )

c Is impaired by hypoproteinaemia. ( )

d Is stimulated by steroids. ( )

58 The principles of wound care include:

a Early skin cover. ( )

b Removal of foreign material. ( )

c Routine administration of antibiotics. ( )

d Close apposition of uninfected wounded tissues. ( )

59 Heavily contaminated and dirty wounds:

a Require surgical toilet and delayed closure. ( )

b Require the administration of systemic antibiotics. ( )

c Can usually be treated by wound toilet and primary closure. ( )

d Should be totally excised. ( )

a **T—** Polymorphs and monocytes accumulate and engulf cell debris and all foreign material during the initial phase of repair.

b **F—** A clean incised wound whose edges are opposed is re-epithelialized within 2 days.

c **F—** Healed skin wounds are never as strong as unwounded skin. After 8 weeks it has reached 80 per cent of its original strength.

d **T—** These cells synthesise collagen.

a **F—** No studies have confirmed this widely held view.

b **T—** Any foreign material, fluid or haematoma prolongs the inflammatory phase and inhibits fibroblast invasion.

c **T—** An albumin concentration below 2.5 g/100 ml significantly impairs wound healing.

d **F—** Steroids decrease the rate of epithelialization and inhibit fibroblast proliferation. They thus have an inhibitory effect on wound healing.

a **T—** The principles of meticulous debridement and careful tissue
b **T** apposition should be adhered to whether the wound is from a sterile
c **F** surgical knife or is the untidy contaminated wound of a road traffic
d **T** accident. Skin grafts should cover skin defects as soon as possible. When wound toilet is not possible within 12 to 18 hours it is usually best to delay closure of the wound because by this time active bacterial multiplication has occurred. Antibiotics should only be used when infection is likely to have occurred.

a **T—** Meticulous removal of dead and foreign material coupled with the
b **T** administration of a suitable broad spectrum antibiotic and gentle
c **F** packing with gauze prior to delayed closure 4 or 5 days later is the most effective form of treatment.
d **F—** The remaining wound would be scarcely less contaminated and such radical therapy is usually only necessary in spreading infections such as gas gangrene.

60   Surgical drainage of abscesses:
a   Should be via a small incision with minimal disturbance of   (   )
the adjacent tissues.
b   Should be dependent wherever possible.   (   )
c   Has been outmoded by antibiotic therapy.   (   )

d   Should be undertaken before the signs of fluctuation appear.   (   )

61   In localised surgical infections:
a   An elevated leucocyte count is usually present.   (   )
b   Fever and tenderness are usually present.   (   )
c   The presence of glycosuria usually indicates metastatic   (   )
pancreatic abscesses.
d   Pus is frequently absent.   (   )

62   Staphylococcal infections:
a   Do not cause cellulitis.   (   )
b   Do not produce septicaemia.   (   )

c   Do not produce fever.   (   )
d   Produce yellow odourless pus.   (   )

63   Streptococcal infections:
a   Are characterised by abscess formation.   (   )
b   Rarely produce lymphadenitis.   (   )
c   Frequently produce bacteraemia.   (   )

d   Can produce a gangrenous skin infection.   (   )

a   F— Bold incisions, with the breaking down of all loculi and the removal of slough should be undertaken.
b   T— Gravity will help drainage.
c   F— Antibiotics are of little value in the treatment of an abscess but when cellulitis surrounds the abscess, they should be used as an adjunct to surgery.
d   F— At this point the infection may be at the cellulitic stage and not localised. It is then justifiable to administer antibiotics and carefully observe the response. (Fluctuation is, of course, only elicited in palpable abscesses.)

a   T— In an infection attenuated by prolonged and partially effective
b   T   antibiotic therapy these common signs are frequently absent.
c   F— Diabetes and infection do however frequently co-exist and make the treatment of each more difficult.
d   F— It is a characteristic of all localised infections that pus (necrotic cellular debris, macrophages and bacteria) is found surrounded by granulation tissue and fibrosis (the abscess wall).

a   F— Staphylococcal cellulitis does occur.
b   F— Septicaemia does occur and may be accompanied by septic shock and metastatic abscess formation.
c   F— Pyrexia is present in all but the smallest skin eruptions.
d   T— This characterises a staphylococcal abscess.

a   F— They are characteristically invasive and produce cellulitis.
b   F— Lymphangitis and lymphadenitis are common.
c   T— This should be suspected when an unexplained pyrexia, rigor or toxaemia develops.
d   T— Streptococcal gangrene, due to anaerobic organisms, is characterised by oedema and haemorrhagic skin bullae. It may be confused with a clostridial cellulitis.

64 **Tetanus prophylaxis in a patient with a badly contaminated wound:**

a Depends, even in an actively immunised patient, on   (   )
meticulous immediate debridement of the wound.

b Should include the administration of tetanus toxoid.   (   )

c Is more safely achieved with equine rather than human   (   )
antitoxin.

d Is unnecessary in patients who have been recently actively   (   )
immunised.

65 **Tetanus:**

a May have an incubation period of over 20 days.   (   )

b Can be prevented by the immediate administration of   (   )
tetanus toxoid.

c Is more common after scalp lacerations than wounds of   (   )
the extremities.

d Is usually associated with stupor or coma.   (   )

66 **The treatment of established tetanus:**

a Should include wound excision.   (   )

b Has been improved by the use of mechanical ventilation.   (   )

c Requires adequate and prolonged antibiotic therapy.   (   )

d Should include treatment with human antitetanus   (   )
antitoxin.

a   **T**– This is ESSENTIAL and cannot be over-emphasised.

b   **T**– The previously unimmunised patient should also receive antitetanus toxin; the actively immunised patient requires a booster dose of toxoid.

c   **F**– The antibody titre remains higher for a longer period with the human antitoxin. The equine variety is complicated by allergic reactions and cross-sensitivity in about half the patients.

d   **F**– See b–prophylaxis should ALWAYS include wound care.

a   **T**– This may vary from 3 to 24 days.

b   **F**– Active immunisation will not confer protection for 2 to 3 weeks after the injection of the toxoid. Wounds which are contaminated with foreign bodies or necrotic tissue are particularly at risk. Prophylaxis should include adequate wound toilet and passive immunisation of the previously unimmunised patient. Patients who have had a full course of active immunisation with toxoid require a booster dose.

c   **F**– Injuries of the extremities are more frequently complicated by tetanus. The rich blood supply of the scalp confers some protection.

d   **F**– The patient's conscious level is rarely depressed.

a   **T**– This will prevent the release of further exotoxins.

b   **T**– The spasms and clonic contractions that characterise the severe infection are painful, distressing and may interfere with respiration. Thus, these cases may need treatment with muscle relaxants, sedatives and mechanical ventilation.

c   **F**– Although antibiotics may be required for the initial treatment of the causative wound, they are ineffective in the treatment of established tetanus.

d   **T**– The human, rather than the equine, antitoxin allows successive doses of antitoxin to be given subcutaneously and systemically. It has improved the results of treatment.

67 **Clostridial myositis:**

a Is otherwise known as gas gangrene. ( )
b Has a 2 to 3 week incubation period. ( )

c May produce jaundice. ( )
d May rapidly produce anaemia. ( )

68 **In clostridial infections:**

a A spreading cellulitis may be present. ( )

b Gram-positive cocci can be isolated from the discharge. ( )
c Surgical treatment has a minor part to play. ( )

d Gas production is often absent. ( )

69 **Actinomycosis is characterised by:**

a Chronic abscesses of the cervico-facial region. ( )
b A granulomatous abscess wall. ( )
c Red coloured pus. ( )

d Its resistance to antibiotics. ( )

70 **A subphrenic abscess:**

a Is usually accompanied by considerable systemic effects. ( )
b Is associated with local rib tenderness. ( )
c Rarely produces abnormal signs in the chest. ( )
d May be diagnosed by a barium meal examination. ( )

a   T— It is caused most frequently by *C.welchii* and *C.septicum*.
b   F— This is a very rapidly progressive infection generally associated with a poor blood supply and delayed surgical care to contaminated wounds.
c   T— The many clostridial exotoxins giving rise to severe systemic effects
d   T   include potent haemolysins.

a   T— *Clostridium welchii* may cause this serious condition. It is characterised by a rapidly spreading crepitant cellulitis.
b   F— Clostridia are gram-positive rod shaped bacilli.
c   F— Early desloughing, wound toilet and surgical decompression by incision and fasciotomy are essential. Antibiotics are an adjunct to surgery.
d   T— *Clostridium tetani* does not generally produce gas and gas production in *clostridium welchii* cellulitis and myositis may be absent. Streptococcal cellulitis and mixed infections sometimes produce gas in the tissues.

a   T— Other common sites are the chest wall and the caecum.
b   T— The fibrotic abscess wall contains many granulomata and tangled
c   F   masses of branching filaments ('sulphur' granules) which give a characteristic yellow colour to the pus.
d   F— The infection can be effectively treated by a 3 to 4 week course of penicillin or tetracycline.

a   F— The signs and symptoms of this condition are frequently minimal, with only a mild pyrexia and a leucocytosis being present. Occasionally there
b   T   is tenderness between the overlying ribs, a sympathetic pleural effusion
c   F   in the adjacent pleural cavity, shoulder tip pain and hiccoughs.
d   T— A left sided subphrenic abscess may be noted on barium meal by indentation of the fundus of the stomach. The most commonly employed radiological technique is to observe diaphragmatic movement under fluoroscopy. This is diminished on the affected side.

71   **A pelvic abscess:**
a   Lies extraperitoneally.   (   )
b   May be a complication of abdominal surgery.   (   )

c   Often presents with diarrhoea.   (   )

d   Should be treated with antibiotics alone.   (   )

72   **Paralytic ileus:**
a   Is associated with electrolyte imbalance.   (   )
b   May be associated with mechanical intestinal   (   )
     obstruction.
c   Requires treatment with nasogastric suction and   (   )
     intravenous fluids.

d   Is associated with retroperitoneal haematoma.   (   )

73   **Acute postoperative gastric dilatation:**
a   May cause postoperative vascular collapse.   (   )

b   Can be prevented by regular nasogastric aspiration.   (   )

c   Characteristically occurs on the first postoperative day.   (   )
d   Is a relatively common problem after surgery on the   (   )
     gastrointestinal tract.

74   **The appearance of jaundice in the postoperative period:**
a   May indicate an intraperitoneal haemorrhage.   (   )

b   Is usually due to the toxic effects of anaesthetic agents.   (   )

c   May be due to septicaemia.   (   )
d   May indicate chronic liver disease.   (   )

a　F—　This abscess lies in the lowest cul-de-sac of peritoneum, the recto-
b　T　vesical or recto-uterine pouch. It may also result from an infected
　　　　neighbouring viscus, e.g. appendix or from generalised peritonitis.
c　T—　Watery diarrhoea frequently results from associated rectal inflammation.
　　　　The systemic effects of an abscess are also present.
d　F—　Antibiotics are useful when the pelvic infection is at the cellulitic stage
　　　　and as an adjunct to surgery. They cannot alone treat an established
　　　　abscess and surgical drainage is required.

a　T—　There are abnormal fluid and electrolyte losses in a patient with
b　T　paralytic ileus. Hypokalaemia particularly contributes to further
　　　　inhibition of intestinal motility by interfering with the normal ionic
c　T　movements during smooth muscle contraction. Prolonged intestinal
　　　　distension such as is associated with mechanical intestinal obstruction
　　　　may also inhibit intestinal motility. Decompression of the distended
　　　　bowel by nasogastric suction and replacement of the abnormal fluid
　　　　losses form the basis of treatment after mechanical causes of the
　　　　obstruction have been ruled out.
d　T—　Retroperitoneal haemorrhage, severe trauma, particularly to the
　　　　vertebral column, and ureteric distension all inhibit intestinal
　　　　motility.

a　T—　Gastric distension (with up to 5 or 6 litres of fluid) is associated with
　　　　hypovolaemia.
b　T—　This is frequently undertaken for the first 2 to 3 postoperative days
　　　　until flatus is passed and bowel sounds return to normal.
c　F—　It usually occurs 2 or 3 days after operation.
d　F—　The routine use of postoperative nasogastric suction has almost
　　　　abolished its incidence after abdominal surgery. It still occurs in severe
　　　　injuries and burns where nasogastric suction is less commonly used.

a　T—　The blood is haemolysed producing a transient mild haemolytic
　　　　jaundice.
b　F—　Certain anaesthetic agents (such as chloroform and possibly halothane)
　　　　have a hepatotoxic effect, but the incidence is very low.
c　T—　Severe sepsis may give rise to jaundice, probably by haemolysis.
d　T—　Hypotension and hypoxia during the operative period may
　　　　precipitate jaundice in a patient with chronic liver disease.

75 **A distal small bowel fistula:**

a Loses intestinal fluid rich in potassium and sodium. ( )

b May give rise to a metabolic acidosis. ( )

c Rapidly results in dehydration. ( )

d May be managed conservatively by the abandonment of oral feeding. ( )

76 **A pancreatic fistula:**

a Loses fluids with high potassium and lower sodium levels than plasma. ( )

b May give rise to a metabolic acidosis. ( )

c Requires long term treatment with intravenous normal saline. ( )

d Will usually close if oral feeding is temporarily suspended. ( )

77 **Bed sores:**

a Can be prevented by sheepskin blankets. ( )

b Can be prevented by changing the patient's position four times each 24 hours. ( )

c Are the consequence of local infection. ( )

d Only occur over the sacrum. ( )

V Skin and Breast

78 **Malignant melanomata:**

a Occur more commonly in the black races. ( )

b Occur with equal frequency in all ages. ( )

c Frequently arise from pre-existing benign naevi. ( )

d Occur more frequently in tropical regions. ( )

a T— The concentration of sodium in the fistulous fluid is comparable to plasma and that of potassium often higher.
b T— This is due to the alkaline nature of the fistulous losses.
c T— Water losses may be as much as 4 or 5 litres per day.
d T— Provided there is no distal obstruction, parenteral nutrition and the cessation of oral feeding may result in a decrease of the fistulous losses and eventual closure.

a F— The sodium and potassium levels in pancreatic fluid are similar to those of plasma.
b T— There are high bicarbonate losses.
c F— Because of b the patient must be sustained on sodium lactate or bicarbonate solution.
d F— The high concentration of enzymes renders skin excoriation a major problem and abandonment of oral feeding will only slightly diminish the volume of fistula losses. It thus has little effect on the healing of the fistula.

a F— Bed sores are due to local ischaemia. This may occur over any bony
b F   prominences, the back of the head, the heels and the greater trochanter of the femur as well as the sacrum. They are often the consequence of
c F   inadequate nursing (and medical) care and observation. They are best
d F   prevented by changing the patient's position every 2 hours. Sheepskin and foam underlays add support to the nursing endeavours.

a F— These are rare in the black races where they are usually found only in the depigmented skin of the feet and hands.
b F— They usually present between the ages of 30 and 60. They are very rare in the prepubertal child.
c T— Approximately half the patients give a history of change in a pre-existing stable pigmented lesion.
d T— The incidence in the white races is related quite closely to the amount of solar radiation received. The highest incidence is in white Australians.

79 **A malignant melanoma:**

a Frequently arises from hair-bearing naevi. ( )

b Frequently arises from junctional naevi. ( )

c Has a worse prognosis when it arises on the leg. ( )

d Should be suspected in any pigmented lesion which bleeds spontaneously. ( )

80 **The treatment of a malignant melanoma should include:**

a A preliminary incision biopsy. ( )

b Wide excision of the tumour. ( )

c 'En bloc' removal of adjacent involved lymph nodes. ( )

d Immediate excision of any enlarging lymph node in the postoperative period. ( )

81 **Squamous cancer of the lip:**

a Is most common in early adult life. ( )

b Is more common in fair skinned subjects. ( )

c Metastasises readily by the blood stream. ( )

d Is preferably treated by radiotherapy once lymph node deposits are present. ( )

a   F— These naevi contain dermal elements and have a very low malignant
        potential.
b   T— These flat, usually darkly pigmented lesions are those most likely to
        undergo malignant change.
c   F— Lower limb melanomata have the best prognosis. Head, neck and trunk
        melanomata have the worst. Late recognition is thought to be a factor
        in explaining the poor survival of the latter group.
d   T— This is a warning sign, together with itching, ulceration, progressive
        growth and increased pigmentation.

a   F— Dissemination by blood and lymphatic systems frequently follows this
        procedure.
b   T— The extent of the excision is related to the size and site of the primary,
        but many authorities state that a 5 cm margin of normal tissue is the
        minimum to be excised.
c   T— But the policy regarding 'prophylactic' lymph node removal when they
        are remote from the tumour and possibly uninvolved is less certain and
        much controversy exists.
d   T— Examinations should be carried out every 1 to 3 months for at least
        the first two years. Enlargement of regional nodes is then noted early
        and is an indication for immediate excision of those nodes. In this way
        systemic spread can be avoided in some patients.

a   F— There is an increasing incidence with age. It is particularly common
b   T   in people exposed to large amounts of sunlight particularly if their
        skin has little natural pigmentation. It is very rare in the black races.
c   F— The most common mode of spread is by direct extension to
        neighbouring tissues. Lymphatic spread does occur, particularly in
        poorly differentiated lesions, but spread via the blood stream is
        uncommon.
d   F— Surgical excision is recommended with block dissection of the neck
        if there is evidence of lymph node metastasis. Radiotherapy on its own
        is indicated for small well-differentiated lesions, when the possibility
        of metastasis is unlikely, or as palliative treatment in the late stages of
        the disease.

82 **Basal cell carcinomas:**
a Usually metastasise to regional lymph nodes. ( )

b Are less common than squamous cell carcinomas. ( )
c Are characterised histologically by epithelial pearls. ( )

d Are particularly common in oriental races. ( )

83 **Capillary angiomas of childhood (strawberry naevi):**
a Arise in the dermis. ( )
b Are premalignant. ( )
c Are most satisfactorily treated with superficial ( )
  radiotherapy.
d Should be surgically excised. ( )

84 **Fibroadenomata of the breast:**
a Are commonest in early adult life. ( )
b Are indiscrete and difficult to distinguish. ( )
c Are usually painless. ( )
d Resolve without treatment. ( )

85 **Fibrocystic disease of the breast:**
a Is a variant of the normal cyclical changes that the breast ( )
  undergoes during menstruation.
b Is normally unilateral. ( )

c Tends to progress in the post-menopausal years. ( )

d Is precancerous. ( )

a   F—   While this is so in squamous cell carcinomata, metastases are very rare in basal cell lesions.

b   F—   They are approximately three times more common.

c   F—   These are characteristic of squamous cell carcinomas. The classical appearance in basal cell lesions is of darkly staining solid masses of cells arising from the basal layer of epidermis.

d   F—   Such lesions are rare in oriental and almost unknown in black races. They typically occur in 'sunworshipping' blonde subjects and on the exposed skin of outdoor workers.

a   T—   They are raised, reddish-purple dermal vascular malformations. They

b   F   have no malignant potential.

c   F—   The vast majority will spontaneously regress by 3 years of age. If this does not occur then a short dose of steroids may initiate regression.

d   F   Radiotherapy for this or any other benign lesion is to be condemned because of the possible dangers of ensuing malignancies. Surgery is rarely necessary. Capillary angiomas should be distinguished from cavernous angiomas which develop from larger vessels. The latter appear in childhood, do not regress and frequently require surgical treatment.

a   T—   The peak incidence is in the third decade.

b   F—   They are firm, smooth, well circumscribed, mobile lumps.

c   T—   In the majority of patients this is so.

d   F—   They tend to enlarge.

a   T—   There is glandular hyperplasia, cyst formation, duct wall hyperplasia, periductal fibrosis and lymphocytic infiltration.

b   F—   It is usually bilateral and most common in the upper outer quadrant of the breasts.

c   F—   Though it is most common in the later years of reproductive life, some regression and decrease in pain occurs after the menopause.

d   F—   There is no conclusive evidence to support this view.

true or false

86   The management of fibrocystic breast disease should:
a   Usually be by surgical excision.   (   )

b   Include mammography when available.   (   )

c   Include therapy with oestrogens.   (   )
d   Include therapy with progesterone.   (   )

87   An intraduct papilloma of the breast:
a   May cause a bloody nipple discharge.   (   )
b   May be diagnosed with the aid of contrast radiography.   (   )

c   Should be treated by simple mastectomy.   (   )

d   Is associated with fibrocystic disease of the breast.   (   )

88   Paget's disease of the nipple:
a   Usually presents as a bilateral eczema of the nipple.   (   )
b   Is always related to an underlying breast cancer.   (   )

c   Indicates incurable breast cancer.   (   )

d   Has non-specific histological characteristics.   (   )

89   X-ray examination of the breast (mammography):
a   Does not improve the clinician's diagnosis rate of benign   (   )
        and malignant breast disease.
b   Is diagnostically most useful in young women.   (   )

c   Is practical as a nationwide presymptomatic screening   (   )
        procedure in the United Kingdom.
d   Contributes nothing to the management of the patients   (   )
        with clinically obvious breast cancer.

a   F—   This is an extremely common condition and the majority of patients are treated symptomatically. Only when the lesion is discrete and carcinoma is suspected is an excision biopsy undertaken.

b   T—   Where this facility exists, advantage should be taken of its ability to distinguish breast cancer from fibrocystic disease. It may also detect a neoplasm whose diagnosis is obscured by surrounding (and unrelated) fibrocystic disease of the breast.

c   F—   These do not influence the progress of the disease although pain relief

d   F   may be achieved, particularly by progesterone.

a   T—   This and the occurrence of pain are the most frequent symptoms.

b   T—   Injection of the relevant duct with contrast medium often confirms the diagnosis.

c   F—   Local removal of this benign lesion with or without segmental resection of the breast is all that is required.

d   F—   This benign neoplasm is not to be confused with the diffuse papillomatous lesions often seen in fibrocystic breast disease.

a   F—   It is usually a unilateral disease.

b   T—   The lesion is an intraduct carcinoma arising in the minute ducts of the nipple. It infiltrates the skin and often extends deeply to produce a palpable mass.

c   F—   There is a good prognosis in these tumours when compared to other breast cancers. This is probably related to earlier diagnosis and treatment.

d   F—   The histology is characteristic, viz: large clear vacuolated cells (Paget's cells) invading the dermis, epidermal hypertrophy and dermal lymphocytic infiltration.

a   F—   The diagnosis rate is improved by 10 to 15 per cent.

b   F—   The active young breast is relatively radio-opaque and the infiltrating opacification and punctate calcification of breast cancer are rendered more difficult to see.

c   F—   The logistic demands of this screening technique, in terms of manpower and equipment, are far too excessive.

d   F—   Mammography may reveal impalpable cancers and thus bilateral cancers will be diagnosed twice as frequently.

90 **Breast cancer:**
a Is the commonest female neoplasm in the United Kingdom. ( )
b Has its highest incidence in social class V. ( )
c Has a familial tendency. ( )

d Is less common in nulliparous women. ( )

91 **Breast cancer:**
a Often presents with a history of breast pain. ( )

b Is most common in the upper outer quadrant of the breast. ( )

c Can be diagnosed preoperatively by the experienced ( )
clinician in 95 per cent of cases.
d Must be considered on discovering any discrete mass in the ( )
breast.

92 **The signs and symptoms of breast cancer include:**
a A milky nipple discharge. ( )
b Eczematous changes in the nipple and areola. ( )

c Pre-menstrual breast pain. ( )
d Skin tethering. ( )

93 **The histological study of breast cancers has shown that:**
a The prognosis is not related to histological type. ( )

b The commonest carcinoma is a squamous carcinoma. ( )
c Most breast cancers arise from the epithelium of the ( )
breast lobule.
d Satellite breast cancers are common. ( )

a   T— Followed by large bowel and uterine cancer.
b   F— The highest incidence is in social class I.
c   T— A maternal history or a history of a sibling with the disease increases
       the incidence of breast cancer up to 15 times that of the general
       population.
d   F— Nulliparous women have the highest incidence of breast cancer,
       followed by those who did not have their first child until 25 years of
       age. Breast feeding seems to confer some slight protection.

a   T— Though a painless lump is the first sign in two-thirds of patients, in
       more than 15 per cent pain is the presenting symptom.
b   T— Half the breast cancer occurs in the upper outer quadrant and only
       5 per cent in the lower inner quadrant. Medial lesions are much less
       common.
c   F— Most studies show clinical diagnosis to be accurate in only 70 per cent
       of cases—thus all discrete non-cystic breast lumps must be subjected to
d   T   biopsy.

a   F— Cancer should be suspected if a nipple discharge is bloodstained.
b   T— Paget's disease of the nipple, which produces eczematous changes in
       the nipple, is always associated with an underlying breast cancer.
c   F— This usually indicates fibrocystic disease of the breast.
d   T— This is best observed in the skin directly over the tumour. Apart from
       cancer only acute inflammation and fat necrosis show this sign.

a   F— Study of untreated patients with breast cancer reveals that the prognosis
       is related to the histological type. The medullary carcinoma, which is
       least invasive, has the best prognosis.
b   F— The vast majority are adenocarcinomata.
c   T— Breast cancers arise from the nipple, the ducts or the lobule epithelium.
       Duct cancer is by far the commonest.
d   T— This is well marked in the commonest tumour—the infiltrating
       adenocarcinoma (scirrhous carcinoma) where early invasion of blood
       and lymph vessels occurs.

94 **Signs of incurable breast cancer include:**
a   Tumour fixity to the chest wall.   (   )
b   Skin ulceration.   (   )

c   Palpably enlarged mobile ipsilateral axillary lymph nodes.   (   )

d   A bloody nipple discharge.   (   )

95 **The incidence of breast cancer:**
a   Increases with age.   (   )
b   Decreases after premenopausal oophorectomy.   (   )

c   Is relatively low in Japan.   (   )

d   Is related to uterine cancer.   (   )

96 **In a patient with breast neoplasia distant metastases may be revealed by:**
a   A radiographic skeletal survey.   (   )
b   A raised serum alkaline phosphatase.   (   )
c   Raised urinary 17—Ketosteroid metabolites.   (   )
d   A raised serum glutamic oxaloacetic transminase (SGOT).   (   )

97 **Palliation of advanced incurable breast cancer:**
a   Can be achieved by oophorectomy in the premenopausal   (   )
    patient.
b   Can be achieved by oestrogen administration in the   (   )
    premenopausal patient.
c   Can be achieved by androgen administration in the   (   )
    postmenopausal patient.
d   Can be achieved by chemotherapeutic agents in pre- and   (   )
    post-menopausal patients.

a T— These two signs together with peau d'orange, lymphoedema of the
b T arm and fixed axillary lymph nodes usually indicate incurable
advanced cancer of the breast.
c F— More than half the enlarged axillary nodes associated with a breast
neoplasm contain no tumour. This may be the result of an immune
response to the tumour.
d F— A bloody discharge may indicate ductal cancer, or invasion of a major
duct by cancer but it need not indicate advanced or incurable disease.

a T— There is an increasing incidence with age after puberty.
b T— Oophorectomy before 40 years of age considerably reduces the
expected incidence.
c T— The incidence in Japan is less than 20 per cent of that in Britain and
the U.S.A.
d F— No causal or associated relationship has been shown to exist.

a T— Although almost half the patients presenting with breast cancer have
b T occult, and at present mostly unidentifiable, metastatic deposits, a
c F careful clinical examination and some routine investigations will
d T reveal some of these deposits. A chest X-ray and a skeletal survey will
reveal some of the chest and bone secondaries, and the serum alkaline
phosphatase and SGOT may be elevated with liver deposits. No serum
urinary factor at present estimated is diagnostic of widespread disease.
It is debatable whether radio-isotope scanning of the bones and liver are
justifiable as a routine measure as yet because of their diagnostic
limitations.

a T— This should be the first procedure to be tried—approximately one third
of patients will respond.
b F— In this group oestrogens often have a stimulatory effect on the cancer.
Oestrogen-containing contraceptive pills are thus contra-indicated.
c T— About 20 per cent of patients will respond.

d T— Single agents such as 5-Fluorouracil and quadruple chemotherapy with
added cyclophosphamide, vincristine and methotrexate have been
shown to produce moderately high remission rates in both groups of
patients.

98   **The prognosis of treated breast cancer:**

a   Is related to the clinical staging of the cancer.   (   )

b   Is related to the number of axillary nodes found to be   (   )
invaded by cancer at operation.

c   Is related to the use of postoperative radiotherapy to the   (   )
regional nodes and operative field.

d   Is better after simple rather than radical mastectomy.   (   )

99   **The prognosis of treated Stage I breast cancer:**

a   Cannot be satisfactorily assessed until 15 years have   (   )
elapsed.

b   Is adversely affected by a subsequent pregnancy.   (   )

c   Is worse in the male.   (   )

d   Is worse if the cancer is discovered during late pregnancy or   (   )
the puerperium.

VI   Thyroid, Parathyroid and Adrenal Glands

100   Signs and symptoms of hyperthyroidism include:

a   Decreased sweating.   (   )

b   An irregular pulse rate.   (   )
c   Cardiac failure.   (   )

d   Diplopia.   (   )

a   T— When treated, approximately 65 per cent of patients with Stage I (Manchester Classification) are alive after 5 years, whereas survival rates of Stage II, III and IV are progressively worse.
b   T— When only 2 or 3 nodes are found to contain tumour and these are removed, survival rates approach those of Stage I. More than 4 affected nodes worsens the prognosis considerably.
c   F— No improvement in longevity following regional radiotherapy as an adjuvant to surgery has been found in patients with breast cancer. Local recurrence of the disease is however diminished.
d   F— Survival and recurrence rates appear to be similar in the various methods of treatment of 'operable' breast cancer. This similarity reflects the inadequacies of clinical staging in that the consequences of occult, unidentified metastases may disguise the small differences between the various methods of treatment.

a   T— The vast majority of recurrent breast neoplasms occur in the first 15 years after treatment. Survival rate after 15 years parallels that of a comparable age group in the general population.
b   F— The survival rate is significantly improved in those patients who become pregnant after treatment for breast cancer (although oestrogens have a deleterious effect in advanced breast neoplasia in this age group).
c   F— Stage for stage, survival rates are similar in the two sexes, but early spread to adjoining tissues renders more male breast cancers surgically incurable.
d   T— The survival rate is about 5 per cent below that of matched groups of non-pregnant patients.

a   F— There is increased sweating, producing the characteristic warm sweaty palms of the thyrotoxic patient.
b   T— Atrial fibrillation is particularly common in the elderly and the
c   T   deleterious effects on the cardiac output may produce cardiac failure in this group of patients.
d   T— Multiple eye signs of this condition include exophthalmos, lid lag and opthalmoplegia, producing the characteristic facies of the severely thyrotoxic patient.

101 **Symptoms of hyperthyroidism include:**
  a   Intolerance to cold. ( )
  b   Increased appetite. ( )
  c   Emotional instability. ( )
  d   Diarrhoea. ( )

102 **Medical therapy of hyperthyroidism:**
  a   Is particularly indicated in the pregnant patient. ( )

  b   Will usually produce a long-lasting remission rate of ( )
       70 to 80 per cent after a 6 month course.
  c   Is occasionally complicated by bone marrow depression. ( )

  d   Depends on the efficacy of the drugs in inhibiting the ( )
       hypothalamic centres which govern thyroid stimulating
       hormone (TSH) release by the pituitary.

103 **Treatment of hyperthyroidism with radioactive iodine:**
  a   Is complicated by the late occurrence of thyroid ( )
       cancer.
  b   Should not be undertaken in patients below the age of 40. ( )

  c   Is frequently complicated by the development of myxoedema. ( )

  d   Is often complicated by a short-lived exacerbation of the ( )
       hyperthyroid state.

104 **The surgical treatment of hyperthyroidism:**
  a   Is commonly followed by hypothyroidism. ( )
  b   Has a high rate of recurrence. ( )
  c   Can be safely effected without preoperative drug therapy. ( )

  d   May be complicated by postoperative high parathormone ( )
       levels.

a **F—** Amongst the host of symptoms, the most characteristic are weight loss
b **T** associated with an increased appetite. There is marked heat intolerance
c **T** and the development of irritability and emotional instability. Diarrhoea
d **T** and dysmenorrhoea may be prominent.

a **F—** These drugs may cross the placental barrier and inhibit fetal thyroid
function. They may also be excreted in breast milk.
b **F—** Recurrence of hyperthyroidism after drug withdrawal occurs in up to
70 per cent of patients.
c **T—** Both propylthiouracil and carbimazole produce agranulocytosis in a
small number of patients. Drug rashes and hepatitis also occur.
d **F—** The thiouracil group of drugs acts by interfering with the organic
binding of iodine; carbimazole by interfering with tri-iodothyronine
synthesis in the gland.

a **F—** Cumulative experience and close study of patients in the 25 years since
the introduction of therapy with radioactive iodine reveals no
b **T** increased risk of neoplasia. It is advisable however to restrict its use to
those patients in the latter half of life.
c **T—** This may not develop for several years after treatment and the incidence
of hypothyroidism seems to vary in different centres. Hypothyroidism
rates of 40 per cent, 10 years after treatment are common and this
fraction appears to increase with the passage of time.
d **F—** The treatment has no stimulant effect on the gland. Its beneficial effects
are not usually seen for a month or two after ingestion of the
radioactive iodine.

a **F—** Postoperative hypothyroidism can be detected in 5 to 10 per cent of
b **F** patients. There is a similar incidence of recurrent thyrotoxicosis.
c **F—** To operate on the hyperthyroid gland is to court the life-threatening
condition of 'thyroid crisis'—acute severe hyperthyroidism. The
patient must be rendered euthyroid preoperatively with antithyroid
drugs and/or beta-blockers such as propanolol.
d **F—** Postoperative hypoparathyroidism occurs in a small proportion of
patients either due to disturbance to the blood supply of the
parathyroids or their inadvertent removal.

105 **A multinodular (adenomatous) goitre:**

a   Is more common in those patients having a deficient iodine ( )
intake.

b   Is usually preceded by a diffuse goitre in early adult life. ( )

c   Is usually a precancerous condition. ( )

d   Is effectively treated with thyroid hormones to prevent ( )
further adenomatous changes.

106 **Auto-immune thyroiditis (Hashimoto's disease):**

a   Characteristically occurs in young females. ( )

b   Often presents with hyperthyroidism. ( )

c   Produces a soft diffuse enlargement of the thyroid gland. ( )

d   Is associated with regional lymph node enlargement. ( )

107 **Hashimoto's disease:**

a   Is often associated with increased levels of circulating ( )
thyroid antibodies.

b   Is characterised by lymphocytic infiltration and fibrosis of ( )
the thyroid gland.

c   Is usually treated by sub-total thyroidectomy. ( )

d   Should be treated by anti-thyroid drugs. ( )

a T— This has given rise to the term 'endemic goitre' for it refers to the high
       incidence of multinodular goitre in those areas low in naturally occurring
       iodine, e.g. Derbyshire in the United Kingdom, Switzerland and the
       Andes.
b T— TSH stimulation, secondary to the iodine deficiency, results initially
       in diffuse hyperplasia. This is followed years later by the development
       of nodules of hyperplastic gland interposed with areas of involution and
       fibrosis.
c F— Although the incidence of thyroid cancer is increased in some areas of
       endemic goitre there is no evidence to suggest a direct relationship
       between multinodular goitre and neoplasia in the United Kingdom.
d T— Thyroid hormone administration suppresses the effect of TSH on the
       adenomatous gland. In the early stages of the disease iodine can halt
       the development of a multinodular goitre from diffuse glandular
       enlargement.

a F— It occurs most frequently in middle aged females.
b T— This is usually mild and short lived and is followed by the development
       of permanent hypothyroidism.
c F— Diffuse enlargement of the gland does occur, but the gland is firm and
       rubbery.
d F— Lymphadenopathy is not a feature of Hashimoto's disease and if
       present should arouse suspicion of thyroid neoplasia.

b T— There is often a raised titre of anti-thyroglobulin antibodies and
       antibodies against thyroid acinar cells.
b T— Fibrosis is a manifestation of the later stages of the disease.

c F— The appropriate treatment is very individual. It is advisable to take an
d F   open thyroid biopsy; pressure on the trachea may demand excision of
        the thyroid isthmus and very occasionally cosmetic considerations
        require a sub-total thyroidectomy. Thyroid hormones usually have to
        be given to combat hypothyroidism.

108   Thyroid cancer:

a   Frequently produces multinodular enlargement of the gland.   (   )

b   Should be diagnosed by preoperative needle biopsy of the   (   )
gland.

c   Can be excluded if there is a localised but soft enlargement   (   )
of the gland.

d   Often produces a bruit over the gland.   (   )

109   Papillary carcinoma of the thyroid:

a   May follow radiation exposure in childhood.   (   )

b   Is a slow growing tumour.   (   )

c   Usually metastasises to lymph nodes.   (   )

d   Is usually a multifocal tumour.   (   )

110   Follicular carcinoma of the thyroid:

a   Is most common in females.   (   )
b   Is most common above the age of 30 years.   (   )

c   Usually metastasises to lymph nodes.   (   )

d   Is associated with a relatively good prognosis in childhood.   (   )

111   Undifferentiated carcinoma of the thyroid:

a   Is most common in females.   (   )
b   Is most common above the age of 60.   (   )
c   Is often thyroid stimulating hormone (TSH) dependent.   (   )
d   Often exhibits independent thyroid hormone production.   (   )

a   F— Whilst cancer occasionally develops in a multinodular goitre the usual signs of thyroid neoplasia are a localised or generalised swelling of the gland.

b   F— It is difficult to diagnose well-differentiated cancers from the small piece of tissue so obtained and spread of cancer along the needle track occasionally occurs.

c   F— Well-differentiated lesions frequently present as soft solitary swellings. All solitary swellings of the gland should have an excision biopsy performed.

d   F— There is no hypervascularity in thyroid cancer.

a   T— This is most marked in cancers appearing before adolescence. A history of irradiation has been noted in 70 per cent of papillary cancers in this age group.

b   T— This is particularly so in young patients where growth of the primary and metastases is slow.

c   T— Whilst this is the most common mode of spread, spread by the blood stream is not uncommon in the older patient.

d   T— This is frequently noted and may represent intraglandular spread.

a   T— As is papillary carcinoma.

b   T— Whereas papillary carcinoma is most common in children and younger adults.

c   F— Though lymphatic spread does occur, spread by the blood stream to bones and lungs is more frequent.

d   T— There is an increased incidence of well-differentiated, well-encapsulated follicular and papillary carcinomas in this age group and they are associated with a good prognosis.

a   F— There is an equal incidence in the two sexes.

b   T— It rarely occurs before this age.

c   F— The histological picture is of sheets of undifferentiated cells with no

d   F   follicular formation. No evidence of hormonal activity or response to hormonal therapy exists in this type of tumour.

112 **The surgical treatment of thyroid cancer:**
a Should be by 'near total' thyroidectomy in the ( )
potentially curable patient.

b Should include block dissection of the neighbouring lymph ( )
nodes whether or not they appear to contain tumour.

c Is most successful in the papillary type of cancer. ( )

d Should be preceded by a therapeutic dose of I^{131} ( )

113 **Recurrent thyroid cancer can effectively be treated by:**
a High doses of I^{131} ( )
b High doses of thyroid hormone. ( )
c External irradiation. ( )
d Chemotherapy. ( )

114 **The earliest symptoms of hyperparathyroidism include:**
a Diarrhoea. ( )
b Polydipsia and polyuria. ( )
c Unexplained weight gain. ( )
d Muscle spasm. ( )

115 **Primary hyperparathyroidism:**
a Is most common in postmenopausal females. ( )

b Is occasionally diagnosed by routine biochemical screening ( )
of patients.

c Should be considered when a patient presents with tetany. ( )

d Can be caused by adenomas or hyperplasia of the glands. ( )

a   T— Many of the tumours are multifocal and only the posterior rim of thyroid tissue (and associated parathyroid glands) on the opposite side of the neck to the primary tumour should be preserved.
b   F— Only node dissection of apparently involved nodes should be attempted.

c   T— The histological type and the presence or absence of invasion are of great significance in determining the outcome after surgical treatment. Long term survival has been frequently recorded in incompletely removed papillary and follicular carcinomata of the thyroid where these are well differentiated, whereas undifferentiated cancers are uniformly fatal whatever the treatment.
d   F— Histological diagnosis may be interfered with. I ^{131} has no part to play in preoperative therapy.

a   T— A therapeutic dose of radioactive iodine is the treatment of choice.
b   T   TSH suppression by means of thyroid hormones is used in well-
c   T   differentiated tumours with good results. External irradiation is of
d   F   value in palliating undifferentiated tumours and lymphomas. There are as yet no reports of satisfactory remission rates being produced by chemotherapy.

a   F— The earliest symptoms are vague and rarely suggest the diagnosis but
b   T   constipation, muscle weakness, anorexia and weight loss together with
c   F   thirst and polyuria are encountered.
d   F

a   T— It is three times more common in females and particularly frequent between 45 and 65 years of age. It is rare in children.
b   T— The rate of recognition has increased since biochemical screening has been introduced. A raised serum calcium, particularly if associated with a low serum phosphate, is a strong pointer to the diagnosis.
c   F— Tetany only occurs with a low serum calcium. The commonest presenting symptoms are vague abdominal and bone pains. Fractures are not uncommon and renal calculi may produce renal or ureteric colic. Thus the adage: hyperparathyroidism equals 'groans, bones and stones'.
d   T— Single adenomata are the most common cause of the condition. Generalised hyperplasia may cause hyperparathyroidism. Carcinoma is very rarely encountered.

116   **Skeletal signs, symptoms and radiological evidence of hyperparathyroidism:**
a   Include demineralisation of the bones. ( )
b   Include bone cysts and osteoclastoma formation. ( )
c   Include spontaneous fractures. ( )
d   Are the most common presenting complaints. ( )

117   **Renal symptoms of hyperparathyroidism:**
a   May be due to renal stones. ( )
b   May be due to nephrocalcinosis. ( )
c   Are frequently those of chronic renal failure. ( )
d   Are associated with hypertension. ( )

118   **Acute adrenal insufficiency:**
a   In the newborn is due to haemorrhage into one or both adrenal glands. ( )
b   In the newborn typically occurs in the second week of life. ( )
c   In the adult usually follows a pneumococcal septicaemia. ( )
d   In the adult is most frequently encountered following bilateral adrenalectomy. ( )

119   **Phaeochromocytomata:**
a   Are tumours of the spinal nerve roots. ( )
b   Are frequently multiple. ( )
c   Characteristically present with a lemon-yellow skin discolouration. ( )
d   Can be effectively managed by long term medical therapy. ( )

a   T— This is a general phenomenon affecting the whole skeleton.
b   T— This is particularly common in the bones of the lower limbs and ribs.
c   T— These indicate advanced and severe hyperparathyroidism.
d   F— The most common presenting signs and symptoms are those referrable to the renal tract.

a   T— Renal stones occur in over half the patients. Nephrocalcinosis is less
b   T   common, about 5 per cent of patients being affected.
c   T— More than 70 per cent of patients have renal damage and this may be severe especially when nephrocalcinosis is present.
d   T— More than 70 per cent of patients have hypertension and in the majority this is associated with renal damage.

a   T— Adrenal apoplexy in the newborn is usually fatal within the first few days of life. Haemorrhage into the glands occurs at birth and is
b   F   possibly precipitated by withdrawal of maternal hormones. The condition is sometimes associated with birth trauma.
c   F— While streptococcal, staphylococcal and pneumococcal septicaemia may all give rise to the Waterhouse-Friderichsen syndrome it is most commonly associated with fulminating meningococcal septicaemia.
d   F— This should be prevented by the routine administration of steroid replacement during and after the operation.

a   F— They arise from chromaffin cells of the adrenal medulla and sympathetic nervous system.
b   T— 40 per cent are multiple.
c   F— The characteristic symptoms are due to intermittent catecholamine release and thus all the symptoms and signs of sympathetic over-activity such as paroxysmal tachycardia, flushing, sweating and palpitations are intermittently produced. Hypertension will eventually become permanent and diabetes is often present.
d   F— Prompt surgical treatment is the rule. During the operation undue handling of the tumour may result in a very serious tachycardia and a dangerous attack of hypertension. These problems are reduced by effective preoperative sympathetic blockade.

120 **In Cushing's syndrome:**

a   There is usually an increased deposition of fat over the face and trunk.   ( )

b   Hypotension and hypokalaemia are frequently present.   ( )

c   There is an increased production of adrenal hormones.   ( )

d   The cause is most frequently an adrenal tumour.   ( )

121 **Cushing's syndrome:**

a   May be due to adrenal cortical hyperplasia, adrenal adenomata or adrenal carcinomata.   ( )

b   May be associated with bronchogenic cancer.   ( )

c   Is effectively treated by total bilateral adrenalectomy even when shown to be pituitary dependent.   ( )

d   Should be managed medically unless complications develop.   ( )

122 **A thyroglossal cyst:**

a   Usually presents in early adult life.   ( )

b   Is a remnant of fifth pharyngeal arch mesoderm.   ( )

c   Should usually be excised with the thyroid cartilage.   ( )

d   Does not move with swallowing.   ( )

123 **Neuroblastomata:**

a   Usually arise in the renal substance.   ( )

b   Are one of the rarest solid tumours of childhood.   ( )

c   Usually metastasise via the blood stream.   ( )

d   Are difficult to distinguish from Wilms' tumours on clinical examination.   ( )

a   T— Facial and truncal adiposity, polycythaemia, diabetes and skin striae are characteristic findings. The serum potassium is invariably high and
b   F   hypertension is common.
c   T— Diagnostic confirmation can be obtained by serum estimations and urinalysis.
d   F— More than half the cases studied show the causative lesion to be in the pituitary. This liberates ACTH and stimulates the adrenals into overactivity.

a   T— These account for approximately half of the patients seen; the remainder are secondary to pituitary overactivity and a few other rare causes (see b).
b   T— Ectopic ACTH may be produced by several neoplasms of which lung is the commonest.
c   T— This is usually successful. There is a high rate of recurrence if a subtotal adrenalectomy is performed.
d   F— There is, as yet, no curative medical treatment and since the patient progressively worsens, surgical treatment is always advised.

a   F— They most frequently appear before adulthood and one-third of them appear before the age of ten years.
b   F— The thyroid develops as a downgrowth from the back of the tongue into the third and fourth pharyngeal arches. A thyroglossal cyst is a remnant along the course of this tract.
c   F— But it is usually necessary to remove the body of the hyoid bone in order to follow, and remove, the tract into the base of the tongue.
d   F— Like the thyroid gland it moves with the larynx in swallowing.

a   F— These are malignancies of the primitive cells of the sympathetic nervous system, consequently they most frequently arise in the adrenals and less commonly in the sympathetic chain.
b   F— They are the commonest solid tumour of infancy.
c   T— This is common and spread to lungs and bones is frequently seen; local lymphatic spread is also usually present.
d   F— Their nodularity and fixity, especially during respiration, usually enable this distinction to be made.

124   Neuroblastomata:

a   Characteristically produce 5-hydroxyindole acetic acid   (   )
    which can be detected in the urine.
b   Rarely metastasise to bone.   (   )
c   Cannot be satisfactorily treated by surgery.   (   )
d   Have a better prognosis in younger patients.   (   )

VII   Oral Cavity, Pharynx and Oesophagus

125   Surgical repair of a cleft lip and palate:

a   Should not be undertaken until the child begins to talk.   (   )
b   Is essential for normal feeding of the child.   (   )
c   Is essential to ensure normal development of speech.   (   )

d   Should frequently be combined with dental prosthetic work. (   )

126   Salivary duct calculi:

a   Produce pain on eating.   (   )

b   Are commonest in the parotid ducts.   (   )
c   Are a common cause of acute parotitis.   (   )

d   Are associated with hypercalcaemic states.   (   )

127   Salivary tumours:

a   Occur most commonly in the parotid gland.   (   )
b   Of the parotid gland producing facial nerve lesions are   (   )
    usually malignant.

c   May appear as palatal swellings.   (   )

d   Are in most cases satisfactorily treated by radiotherapy.   (   )

a	F—	Most tumours secrete detectable amounts of noradrenaline precursors, e.g. 3-methoxy-4-mandelic acid (VMA).
b	F—	Bone deposits are found in 30 to 40 per cent of patients.
c	F—	Radical surgery is the basis of treatment. In recent years postoperative
d	T	radiotherapy and routine use of vincristine and cyclophosphamide have each been shown to improve survival rates. Spontaneous regression of metastases occasionally occurs. Cure rates of 25 per cent for abdominal neuroblastomata and of 50 per cent (if the child is less than 1 year old) have been reported.

a	T—	Early closure of the defeats is desirable whatever their form; cleft lips
b	T	at about 3 months and palates at 9-12 month. In this way suckling
c	T	difficulties are overcome, there is a likelihood of normal voice development and cosmetic deformities are minimised.
d	T—	Bilateral palatal clefts often require staged surgical correction and an occlusive dental palatal plate may allow normal voice development.

a	T—	The increased production of salivary juice produces painful distension of the gland.
b	F—	The submandibular salivary duct is far more commonly affected.
c	F—	The common causes of acute parotitis are debility, dehydration and poor oral hygiene.
d	F—	There is no evidence that generalised metabolic disorders play any part in the formation of salivary duct calculi. Their aetiology is obscure but may be related to a disturbance in the pH of the saliva.

a	T—	75 per cent of all salivary gland tumours occur in the parotid.
b	T—	The majority of parotid tumours are benign (and of these, the commonest is the mixed parotid tumour) but malignancy is likely if there is an associated facial nerve palsy, an infiltration of the overlying skin or cervical lymph node enlargement.
c	T—	The small and numerous salivery glands of the palate may become neoplastic—the commonest tumour being the highly malignant cylindroma.
d	F—	Surgical excision is the basis of treatment—together with removal of any associated involved nodes.

128 **Cancer of the tongue:**
a Is usually an adenocarcinoma.   (   )

b Is more common in males.   (   )

c Most commonly presents as an indolent ulcer.   (   )

d Metastasises via the lymphatics at an early stage of the   (   )
   disease.

129 **Pharyngeal pouches:**
a Usually occur at the pharyngo-oesophageal junction.   (   )

b Are commonest in young people.   (   )
c May cause pulmonary problems.   (   )

d Usually require surgical excision.   (   )

130 **Pharyngo-oesophageal diverticula:**
a Only occur at the level of cricopharyngeus.   (   )
b May be related to para-oesophageal lymph nodes.   (   )

c Are often associated with recurrent attacks of pneumonitis.   (   )

d Characteristically present with vomiting.   (   )

131 **The diagnosis of oesophageal achalasia may be made by:**
a Oesophageal biopsy.   (   )

b Barium swallow X-ray examination.   (   )

c Oesophagoscopy.   (   )
d Oesophageal motility studies.   (   )

a　F—　Though adenocarcinomas do occur, more than 95 per cent of tongue cancers are of squamous origin.

b　T—　It occurs four times as frequently in males. There is often a history of chronic irritation, leukoplakia, chronic alcoholism or longstanding iron deficiency anaemia.

c　T—　Infiltrative forms of the cancer are recognised but the commonest presentation is of a chronic painless ulcer.

d　T—　More than half the patients have lymph node deposits at the time of presentation and, with cancers of the dorsum of the tongue, these may be bilateral. Surgical excision of the primary tumour and affected lymph nodes forms the basis of treatment. On occasions this is supplemented with radiotherapy.

a　F—　The commonest site is to the left of the midline posteriorly, between the oblique fibres and the transverse cricopharyngeal portion of the inferior constrictor muscle of the pharynx.

b　F—　The majority occur in elderly patients.

c　T—　Aspiration of the diverticular contents may occur, particularly at night, producing aspiration pneumonitis. In addition, dysphagia and gurgling during deglutition may be present.

d　T—　Excision of the diverticulum and closure of the pharyngeal wall is the usual method of treatment.

a　F—　There are three common sites of occurrence, at the level of

b　T　cricopharyngeus, just above the diaphragm, and in the mid-oesophageal region.

c　T—　Aspiration of oesophageal contents is a consequence of the larger diverticula. This occurs particularly at night.

d　F—　Regurgitation, noisy eating and dysphagia are the commonest symptoms.

a　F—　The neurological changes lie submucosally and a deep biopsy would be needed. This is a dangerous procedure.

b　T—　The characteristic finding is of a dilated oesophagus narrowing down in a conical fashion to a smooth stenosis of the cardia.

c　T—　This will distinguish early achalasia from a benign stricture or cancer.

d　T—　In advanced cases there is no peristalsis and no swallowing reflex present. The oesophagus empties purely by gravity.

132   In oesophageal achalasia:

a   Dysphagia is usually the first symptom.   (   )

b   Pain is rarely a prominent symptom.   (   )

c   There is an absence of peristalsis in the oesophagus.   (   )

d   There is an absence of ganglion cells in Auerbach's plexus   (   )
     in the wall of the oesophagus.

133   The treatment of oesophageal achalasia:

a   Is usually by a cardiomyotomy (Heller's operation).   (   )

b   Should primarily be by dilatation.   (   )

c   Should be by oesophagogastrectomy.   (   )

d   Should include a transthoracic vagotomy.   (   )

134   'Sideropaenic dysphagia':

a   Is associated with koilonychia and atrophic oral mucosa.   (   )
b   Is related to longstanding Vitamin B_{12} deficiency.   (   )

c   Is also known eponymously as the 'Paterson-Kelly   (   )
     syndrome' or the 'Plummer-Vinson syndrome'.
d   Is usually due to an oesophageal cancer.   (   )

135   Sliding hiatus herniae:

a   Are associated with a dilated diaphragmatic hiatus.   (   )

b   Are usually readily reducible.   (   )

c   Are usually asymptomatic.   (   )

d   Occasionally strangulate.   (   )

a   T— This is often more marked for liquids than solids, and is eased by
       'trick' swallowing manoeuvres by the patient.
b   F— In more than 25 per cent of cases the patient complains of diffuse
       retrosternal pain in the early stages of the disease. This decreases as
       the functional obstruction worsens.
c   T— The oesophagus is immobile, dilated and empties only by gravity
       through a lower oesophageal sphincter which does not relax
       (cardiospasm).
d   T— Whether this is a primary or secondary phenomenon is not known, but
       it is present in the majority of cases.

a   T— The vast majority of patients are helped by this procedure though
       postoperative reflux oesophagitis may occasionally be a problem.
b   F— Only the relatively mild early cases can be dealt with in this way.
       Oesophageal perforation is an occasional complication of this procedure.
c   F— This is too extensive a procedure and is not rational since the stomach
       is free of any pathology.
d   F— Section of the vagus has no effect on oesophageal motility.

a   T— The majority of cases occur in middle aged or elderly women.
b   F— The majority of cases are associated with long standing iron deficiency
       anaemia. The reason for this association is obscure.
c   T— It was first described in 1919 by Paterson and Kelly.

d   F— The commonest cause is a fibrous web occurring in the upper
       oesophagus. However, about 10 per cent of patients develop cancers
       of the oesophagus, pharynx or oral cavity.

a   T— The cardiac portion of the stomach herniates into the mediastinum
       through a dilated hiatus.
b   T— The oesophagogastric junction will return to the abdomen very readily
       unless oesophageal ulceration or stricture has resulted in shortening of
       the oesophagus.
c   T— Incidental asymptomatic sliding hiatus herniae are frequently
       demonstrated by radiologists.
d   F— These herniae, though not always reducible, have a wide neck at the
       diaphragmatic hiatus and do not strangulate.

136 The symptoms of peptic oesophagitis:
a Include intermittent dysphagia. ( )

b Are often associated with those of anaemia. ( )

c Include retrosternal discomfort. ( )

d Are more likely to occur when the patient is in the upright position. ( )

137 Peptic oesophagitis:
a Is effectively demonstrated by a barium swallow and meal. ( )

b Can be readily confirmed by oesophagoscopy. ( )

c Is associated with the production of higher than normal amounts of gastric acid. ( )

d Is a condition confined to adults. ( )

138 The successful medical management of peptic oesophagitis:
a Should include anticholinergic drugs. ( )
b Includes weight reduction. ( )
c Includes elevating the head of the bed. ( )

d Depends on regular antacid administration. ( )

a   T— Severe oesophagitis produces mucosal oedema and spasm of the underlying oesophageal muscle. This is often intermittent. Submucosal inflammatory changes may eventually produce fibrosis and a stricture of the lower end of the oesophagus. This is often associated with an alleviation of the symptoms of oesophagitis since reflux occurs less readily through the stricture.

b   T— Chronic blood loss may occur from the inflamed and haemorrhagic oesophageal mucosa.

c   T— Retrosternal discomfort is the commonest symptom but discomfort also may be produced in the neck, chest and epigastrium.

d   F— This position often relieves the discomfort, which is usually produced by stooping and lying down.

a   F— Though radiologists are often successful at demonstrating a sliding hiatus hernia, it is known that only some of these patients will have oesophagitis. Oesophagitis may also occur without a hernia being demonstrated. The radiological demonstration of oesophagitis is not usually possible unless spasm or stenosis exists.

b   T— This is the most important investigation. The inflamed mucosa can be recognised by its friability and by contact bleeding. Occasionally ulceration of the mucosa will be seen.

c   F— No relationship between acid output and oesophagitis has been demonstrated. It may be that bile salts are the noxious constituents of the fluid reflux. There is no association with duodenal ulceration.

d   F— Infants born with a congenital hiatus hernia suffer from reflux and oesophagitis.

a   F— Measures to reduce gastric acid secretion are not helpful.

b   T— Weight reduction may reduce intra-abdominal pressure but it only

c   T   alleviates the symptoms slightly. Elevation of the head of the bed is worthwhile, especially in patients with mild symptoms. Regular small meals and reduction in smoking are also of benefit.

d   T— They provide symptomatic relief and may reduce reflux by increasing the tone of the gastro-oesophageal sphincter.

139   Surgical management of peptic oesophagitis:

a   Is indicated in the majority of patients.   (   )

b   Is based on the prevention of reflux.   (   )

c   Is best restricted to repeated bouginage when peptic   (   )
     strictures are present.

d   Should include a vagotomy.   (   )

140   Paraoesophageal hiatus herniae:

a   Usually occur through a defect in the diaphragm to the right   (   )
     of the oesophagus.

b   Usually have an easily recognised hernial sac.   (   )

c   Are usually accompanied by oesophagitis.   (   )

d   May produce postprandial chest pain.   (   )

141   Paraoesophageal hiatus herniae:

a   Are frequently associated with gastric ulceration.   (   )

b   Are frequently accompanied by occult gastrointestinal blood   (   )
     loss.

c   Are congenital in origin.   (   )

d   Should be managed conservatively in the majority of   (   )
     patients.

142   Cancer of the oesophagus:

a   Usually presents with intermittent dysphagia.   (   )

b   Has its highest incidence in the 5th decade.   (   )

c   Is reliably diagnosed by barium swallow.   (   )

d   Should be assessed endoscopically when surgical resection is   (   )
     contemplated.

a   F—   The necessary surgical procedure involves a major abdominal or thoracic operation. It has a significant morbidity and a small mortality. Only incapacitating symptoms are an indication for surgery.

b   T—   Several surgical procedures exist and their rationale is, in all cases, the prevention of reflux.

c   F—   Bouginage will provide only short-term relief. It permits reflux to recur with the recurrence of oesophagitis. Bouginage combined with surgical prevention of reflux is, however, very satisfactory management.

d   F—   Reducing gastric acid secretion has a minimal effect on oesophagitis.

a   F—   The hernial ring is always on the left side of the oesophagus.

b   T—   These are true herniae of the fundus of the stomach into the chest. The cardia remains in its usual abdominal position.

c   F—   There is not usually any incompetence of the cardia so reflux of gastric contents and oesophagitis does not occur.

d   T—   The distension of the intrathoracic portion of the stomach after meals produces a severe 'crushing' pain in the chest and this is often confused with angina.

a   T—   Ulceration of the portion of the stomach inside the hernia is common.

b   T—   Bleeding occurs from gastric ulceration or the area of gastritis which is frequently present in the part of the stomach adjacent to the hernial ring.

c   F—   They are rarely seen before middle age and are most common in the elderly. It is generally assumed they are acquired lesions.

d   F—   Treatment is usually surgical and is often indicated because of the distressing symptoms, the chronic blood loss and the risk of strangulation or perforation.

a   F—   The commonest symptom is a progressive unremitting dysphagia.

b   F—   The incidence rises with age and is most common in patients over 70.

c   T—   Positive information is yielded by this investigation in more than 95 per cent of patients.

d   T—   This allows biopsy or cytological examination of the lesion by oesophagoscopy. Bronchoscopy should be performed to establish whether the trachea or bronchi are invaded by tumour.

true or false

143 **Malignant tumours of the oesophagus:**
a   Are most commonly adenocarcinomas.   (   )

b   Occur most commonly in males.   (   )

c   Are most commonly situated in its upper third.   (   )

d   Commonly spread by lymphatics.   (   )

144 **In the treatment of oesophageal cancers:**
a   Surgical excision of the tumour is feasible in the majority of   (   )
    patients.
b   Radiotherapy is frequently used.   (   )

c   Chemotherapy is of particular value in squamous cell   (   )
    lesions.
d   Gastrostomy provides good palliation for patients with   (   )
    complete dysphagia.

145 **Vomiting against a closed glottis:**
a   May cause a 'spontaneous' rupture of the oesophagus.   (   )
b   May be followed by severe chest pain and circulatory   (   )
    collapse.

c   May cause a laceration of the mucosa of the oesophagogastric   (   )
    junction.
d   May cause gastrointestinal bleeding.   (   )

76

a F— The squamous cell carcinoma is by far the commonest tumour.
        Adenocarcinomas are almost entirely confined to the lower end of the
        oesophagus where they arise from the columnar epithelium adjacent to
        the cardia.
b T— Overall, these malignancies are between 2 and 5 times more frequent in
        males, although cancers of the upper third of the oesophagus occur
        predominantly in females.
c F— About half the malignancies occur in the middle third and about one
        third in the lower third.
d T— Intramural extension, spread to lymph nodes and local spread to
        invade adjacent structures are all very common. Blood borne metastases
        are rare.

a F— The resectability rate is usually less than 30 per cent because of its
        frequent spread to other mediastinal structures.
b T— The squamous cell carcinoma is radiosensitive. Thus, radiotherapy
        finds a place in palliation of inoperable cases, as an adjunct to surgery
        pre- and post-operatively and as a sole means of therapy (particularly
        in upper third cancers).
c F— No chemotherapeutic agents have been shown to be useful in the
        treatment of oesophageal neoplasia.
d F— Gastrostomy will not relieve this symptom. Complete dysphagia
        demands early palliation to relieve the distressing symptoms of
        constantly drooling saliva. Radiotherapy or insertion of a tube through
        the tumour are more effective.

a T— There is a rapid increase in intraluminal pressure which may be
b T   followed by rupture of the lower end of the oesophagus with expulsion
        of air and gastric contents into the mediastinum and pleural cavity
        (usually the left side). This condition is known as the Boerhaave
        syndrome after the name of the first recorded patient. Immediate
        surgical repair is required. The mortality is high.
c T— This is known as the 'Mallory-Weiss' syndrome. There is no pain
        associated with the bleeding; barium studies are not as helpful as
d T   endoscopy in diagnosis. Surgical measures are occasionally required to
        stop continuing bleeding.

VIII   Trachea and Thorax

146   **The airway of an unconscious patient:**
a   Is protected from aspiration of vomit in the semiprone   (   )
position.
b   Is especially at risk in injuries of the face and neck.   (   )
c   Can be effectively protected from vomit by an oropharyngeal   (   )
tube.
d   Can be effectively protected from aspiration of vomit by a   (   )
cuffed endotracheal tube.

147   **The indications for a tracheostomy include:**
a   Sputum retention.   (   )
b   An inadequate tidal volume.   (   )
c   A flail chest.   (   )
d   Tetanus.   (   )

148   **The complications of a tracheostomy include:**
a   Laryngeal stenosis.   (   )

b   Erosion of the left brachiocephalic vein.   (   )
c   Erosion of the innominate artery.   (   )

d   Tracheoesophageal fistula.   (   )

149   **A flail chest wall segment in an injured patient:**
a   Demands that frequent blood gas analysis is undertaken.   (   )
b   Does not usually require mechanical ventilation.   (   )

c   Should be treated by skeletal fixation.   (   )

d   Is frequently complicated by myocardial or pulmonary   (   )
contusion.

a   T— In the 'first aid' situation the positioning of the patient head down and semiprone protects him from aspiration.

b   T— Because of the possibility of direct trauma to the airway.

c   F— Although this is a simple method of establishing an airway, it does not protect against aspiration.

d   T— This is the most effective method of protecting the airway in the unconscious and severely injured patient.

a   T— Whenever respiratory function is disturbed by sputum retention which

b   T   is resistant to normal physiotherapeutic manoeuvres, or by an

c   T   inadequate tidal volume (because of fatigue or insufficient stability

d   T   of the chest wall), an elective tracheostomy will allow spontaneous respiration to be more effective by diminishing the dead space and allowing effective bronchial toilet. Assisted respiration will be required in patients with a flail chest (see Q.149) and in those in whom relaxants are being used.

a   F— Tracheal stenosis is usually the result of pressure necrosis and inflammation. It can be avoided by careful attention to cuff pressure and the position of the tracheostomy tube.

b   T— Particularly in children when the vein may be in the root of the neck.

c   T— Especially in children when a cuffed tube may erode through the thin-walled trachea into the artery.

d   T— This is rare, but the likelihood of this complication increases with the time that a cuffed tube is *in situ*.

a   T— Respiration is embarrassed by a flail segment and all except very

b   F   minor degrees of unstable chest wall require respiratory support with positive pressure ventilation through a cuffed endotracheal tube or tracheostomy. There is thus a need for frequent gas analysis.

c   F— Surgical attempts to stabilise the chest have generally been superseded by the use of positive pressure ventilation.

d   T— Myocardial contusion may show ECG changes of a traumatic myocarditis 3 to 4 days post injury. Pulmonary contusion is demonstrable radiologically after 24 hours.

150 **The physical signs associated with crush injuries of the chest include:**
a Pulsus paradoxus. ( )

b Subconjunctival haemorrhage. ( )

c Cardiac arrhythmias. ( )

d Surgical emphysema. ( )

151 **Blunt injuries to the chest:**
a May cause aortic dissection. ( )

b May produce a flail segment of the chest wall. ( )

c May, by causing a flail chest wall segment, embarrass expiration. ( )

d When non-penetrating cannot produce a pneumothorax. ( )

152 **Open chest wounds:**
a Need an immediate thoracotomy. ( )
b Need immediate sealing by any available method. ( )
c Produce mediastinal 'flap'. ( )
d Produce mediastinal shift. ( )

153 **A pulmonary contusion:**
a Is most evident radiologically 1 to 2 days after an injury. ( )
b Does not usually resolve for 3 weeks. ( )
c Does not produce hypoxaemia. ( )
d May require positive pressure ventilation. ( )

a T— This is most likely after severe crush injuries over the sternum when pericardial or myocardial damage results in haemorrhage into the pericardial cavity and cardiac tamponade.

b T— Severe crush injuries to the chest cause acute expulsion of blood from the thoracic cavity. Cervicofacial stasis which is recognisable as a swollen blotchy appearance, together with ecchymoses, is then noticed in the upper trunk, head and neck.

c T— These are common after any injury affecting mediastinal structures. Atrial fibrillation is probably the commonest.

d T— Air may leak into the tissues of the mediastinum or chest wall from a damaged lung or bronchus.

a T— This may be diagnosed by noting unequal pulses in the upper limbs. Occasionally aortic rupture occurs and should be suspected if there is X-ray evidence of widening of the mediastinum. It requires urgent surgery with the use of cardiopulmonary bypass.

b T— When several ribs are fractured in two or more places the stability of a segment of the chest wall is impaired.

c F— Inspiration is hindered because paradoxical movement (inwards on inspiration) of the flail segment prevents the full development of a negative intrathoracic pressure.

d F— Lacerations of the lungs or bronchi can be produced by sudden deceleration or by rib fractures.

a F— The first priority is to seal the wound by any method. This is followed
b T   by resuscitation and then an exploratory thoracotomy.
c T— On inspiration there is shift of the mediastinum towards the uninjured
d T   side which impairs lung function. On expiration the mediastinum moves back towards the injured side.

a T— The initial chest X-ray will often not show the extent of the contusion.
b F— Resolution is complete in about 1 week.
c F— Larger contusions do embarrass respiratory function and produce
d T   hypoxaemia. Mechanical respiratory support is sometimes required.

154 **The diagnosis of haemothorax:**
a Is more easily made on a supine than an erect chest X-ray. ( )

b Cannot be made radiologically until more than 400 ml ( )
blood are present.
c May require needle aspiration of the chest. ( )
d Once confirmed means that conservative measures can be ( )
adhered to.

155 **A spontaneous pneumothorax:**
a Is usually the result of pulmonary tuberculosis. ( )
b Frequently occurs in patients with pre-existing pulmonary ( )
disease.

c Is usually treated without major surgery. ( )
d Usually requires an exploratory thoracotomy. ( )

156 **In a pleural effusion:**
a 500 ml of fluid may not be clinically or radiologically ( )
apparent.

b Needle biopsy of the pleura provides a diagnosis of the ( )
cause in more than 90 per cent of cases.
c Rapid withdrawal of fluid is advisable in the case of large ( )
effusions.

d Blood staining usually indicates an inflammatory pathology. ( )

a F— The supine film allows the blood to spread more thinly and it is easily missed on this view. Lateral and oblique views are more informative.

b T— Even with oblique views quantities smaller than this may be missed.

c T— This should be considered whenever the diagnosis is uncertain.

d F— Blood in the pleural cavity usually leads to the development of an organised thrombus and a fibrothorax. Adequate drainage (possibly by thoracotomy) is therefore usually necessary.

a F— More than 80 per cent occur in non-tuberculous patients and of these
b T   more than half have no obvious pulmonary pathology. Emphysema, bronchitis, bronchiectasis, tuberculosis and neoplasms are the usual causes of the remainder.

c T— Most small pneumothoraces may be treated conservatively. Should the
d F   air leak continue to increase or embarrass pulmonary function then water-sealed intercostal catheter drainage may be required for a few days. Thoracotomy is only required for recurrent pneumothoraces and is advised in order to diagnose and repair, by resection or over-sewing the diseased area of lung, or by pleurectomy.

a T— This quantity of fluid is the minimum necessary to obliterate the costophrenic angles as seen in an erect chest X-ray. Smaller amounts may occasionally be detected radiologically when loculated in an interlobar fissure or between the visceral and parietal pleura.

b F— This diagnostic procedure is only 50 per cent successful. Thus open biopsy of the visceral and parietal walls of the cavity may be necessary.

c F— Rapid withdrawal of large amounts of fluid (over 1500 ml) may precipitate acute unilateral pulmonary oedema. Careful clinical and radiological localization of the fluid is necessary. Once the fluid has been located with the exploring needle, this should be carefully maintained in position throughout the procedure.

d F— The commonest cause of a blood stained effusion is an underlying bronchogenic carcinoma.

157 **In pulmonary tuberculosis:**

a   The primary focus is usually in a lymph node.   (   )

b   The primary focus usually heals completely.   (   )

c   The lesion is charcterised histologically by the Reed-   (   )
Sternberg giant cell.

d   Fibrosis is rare in the late stages of the disease.   (   )

158 **Bronchial adenomas:**

a   Are usually carcinoids.   (   )

b   Are usually cylindromata.   (   )

c   Are liable to become malignant in 10 per cent of cases. (   )

d   Do not usually produce symptoms.   (   )

159 **Adenocarcinoma of the bronchus:**

a   Is equally common in the two sexes.   (   )

b   Is closely associated with pipe smoking.   (   )

c   Has often spread into the pulmonary veins by the time of   (   )
diagnosis.

d   Accounts for 25 per cent of bronchogenic carcinomas.   (   )

160 **In carcinoma of the bronchus:**

a   The overall 5 year survival is 25 per cent.   (   )

b   The overall 5 year survival is 15 per cent.   (   )

c   The mean survival of the inoperable group of patients is   (   )
6 to 8 months.

d   The mean survival of the inoperable group of patients is   (   )
18 to 24 months.

a   F— The primary (Gohn) focus occurs in the periphery of the lung. It is often accompanied by hilar node involvement.
b   T— In a few cases, particularly in the first few years of life, widespread blood stream dissemination occurs to produce miliary tuberculosis.
c   F— The tubercle consists of an area of central necrosis surrounded by epithelioid cells and multinuclear Langerhan's giant cells.
d   F— This is the characteristic finding in the late stages of the disease.

a   T— About 90 per cent are carcinoid and about 8 per cent cylindromata.
b   F   The carcinoid tumour may give rise to the carcinoid syndrome.
c   T— But bronchial adenomas are much less common than bronchogenic cancer (ratio 1 : 50).
d   F— Haemoptysis is the usual presenting complaint but more than half the patients demonstrate bronchiectasis. Occasionally a lung abscess will result from bronchial obstruction.

a   F— It is twice as common in men as in women (squamous and undifferentiated carcinomas are more than 8 times commoner in males than in females).
b   F— The close relationship of cigarette smoking with squamous and undifferentiated forms of bronchogenic carcinoma is less obvious with adenocarcinoma. There is no certain evidence linking pipe and cigar smoking with lung cancer.
c   T— Owing to it being found most frequently in the periphery of the lung, it is often diagnosed late when both lymphatic and blood stream spread has taken place.
d   F— This cancer accounts for only 10 per cent of all bronchogenic cancers. The majority are divided between the squamous and undifferentiated forms.

a   F— Although a 30 per cent 5 year survival rate may be obtained after
b   F   complete removal, only 25 per cent of cases are operable and the overall 5 year survival is in the region of 8 per cent.
c   T— Survival in this group is little affected by palliative surgery, chemotherapy or radiotherapy, although these measures may provide
d   F   some symptomatic relief.

161 **In the diagnosis of carcinoma of the bronchus:**
  a   Sputum cytology gives 3 per cent false positive results.   (   )

  b   Biopsy of an undifferentiated growth is often accompanied   (   )
      by brisk haemorrhage.
  c   Bronchoscopy is diagnostic in 30 to 40 per cent of patients.   (   )

  d   Mediastinoscopy permits examination of both sides of the   (   )
      tracheal bifurcation.

162 **In Pancoast's syndrome:**
  a   The right vocal cord is commonly paralysed.   (   )

  b   Collateral veins develop over the anterior chest wall.   (   )

  c   Nocturnal pain in the upper arm is common.   (   )

  d   The growth is usually an adenocarcinoma of the lung.   (   )

163 **In carcinoma of the bronchus:**
  a   The commonest group of symptoms are due to superadded   (   )
      infection.
  b   The commonest non-metastatic extrapulmonary sign is   (   )
      pulmonary osteodystrophy.
  c   Antidiuretic hormone may be released by the tumour.   (   )

  d   Posterior lateral column degeneration is the commonest   (   )
      spinal cord manifestation.

a   F—   False positives are very rare but the diagnostic yield in all but the most experienced laboratories is not high. Therefore, negative results do not exclude cancer.

b   F—   The bronchial adenoma is notorious for its vascularity and frequently causes troublesome bleeding after biopsy.

c   T—   This investigation allows biopsy of a lesion and the taking of brushings and washings from the bronchial tree. It should preferably be combined with bronchography. It is also very valuable in assessing the operability of the tumour.

d   F—   Although this investigation is a most useful one in assessing operability of a tumour and the extent of nodal involvement in the mediastinum, the examination is largely limited to the right side, by the presence of the aortic arch on the left.

a   F—   The syndrome is produced by involvement of the lower part of the brachial plexus and sympathetic chain by an apical lung neoplasm. Typically there is no vagal or recurrent nerve involvement.

b   F—   Superior vena caval obstruction caused by malignant mediastinal nodes is seen frequently in carcinoma of the bronchus and is not necessarily associated with an apical lung neoplasm or the Pancoast syndrome.

c   T—   Characteristic of this particular tumour is the development of continuous severe pain over the ulnar aspect of the upper limb, the shoulder and the jaw.

d   F—   The commonest tumour is a squamous or an undifferentiated bronchogenic cancer.

a   T—   These give rise to frequent difficulty in the differential diagnosis, particularly with viral infections which are slow to resolve.

b   T—   Quite frequently the first sign to appear is the sudden onset of finger clubbing.

c   T—   This results in fluid retention and a fall in the serum sodium concentration. Cushing's syndrome is, however, the most common endocrine manifestation of this tumour.

d   T—   Cerebral and cerebellar degeneration and peripheral neuropathy also occur.

164 **Malignant neoplasms of the pleura:**
a   Are usually of epithelial origin.   (   )

b   May be associated with finger clubbing.   (   )

c   Are the commonest cause of chylothorax.   (   )

d   Can frequently be cured by surgical treatment.   (   )

165 **Pulmonary embolism:**
a   Can be demonstrated at post mortem in 60 per cent of   (   )
     people over the age of 60.

b   Can usually be diagnosed by a plain chest X-ray.   (   )

c   Of the paradoxical variety has the red and white laminae of   (   )
     the originating thrombus in the reverse of the normal
     order.
d   Can be effectively treated by infusion of streptokinase   (   )
     through a pulmonary artery catheter.

IX   Hernia, Peritoneum and Abdominal Trauma

166 **The diagnosis of an inguinal hernia:**
a   In infants often depends on the history given by its mother.   (   )

b   In the adult is most easily made with the patient in the   (   )
     sitting position.
c   Depends on the hernial sac or cough impulse being felt   (   )
     below the inguinal ligament.

d   Is supported by the presence of a transilluminable scrotal   (   )
     swelling.

a   F— The commonest primary pleural tumours are mesotheliomata. These are neoplasms of connective tissue origin and are believed to be related to asbestos inhalation.
b   F— Arthralgia, fever and finger clubbing are seen in association with localised relatively benign mesotheliomata but not typically with malignant pleural tumours.
c   F— Chylothorax is almost always the result of indirect violence to the chest or surgical trauma. It is occasionally the result of malignant infiltration of the thoracic duct.
d   F— Long term survival of more than two years has not been recorded in any patient with a mesothelioma. Neither surgery, radiotherapy nor chemotherapy appear to influence the course of the disease.

a   T— This remarkably high incidence corresponds to the incidence of clinically silent episodes of lower leg thrombosis demonstrated in this age group by the I^{125} labelled fibrinogen technique.
b   F— Changes are often absent or minimal. A lung scan is helpful and a pulmonary artery angiogram diagnostic.
c   F— A paradoxical embolus is an embolus arising from the lower limb which enters the systemic circulation through a patent foramen ovale and produces arterial occlusion.
d   T— This method of local administration of streptokinase has been effective in producing rapid resolution of the embolus. It has largely superseded the need to perform emergency pulmonary embolectomy.

a   T— An inguinal lump may have been noted only when the child is crying, therefore an isolated examination may not reveal it. A slight thickening of the spermatic cord caused by the empty hernial sac may be palpable.
b   F— The patient should have his groin inspected and palpated when standing.
c   F— Inguinal herniae are seen and felt to emerge through the superficial inguinal ring above the inguinal ligament, femoral herniae are found below it.
d   F— A hernia is not usually transilluminable (whereas epididymal cysts and hydrocoeles usually are).

167 **Inguinal herniae:**
a   In children are usually of the indirect type.   (   )
b   Of the indirect type are congenital in origin.   (   )
c   Will regress spontaneously in children.   (   )
d   In young adults are most commonly of the direct type.   (   )

168 **Strangulated contents of hernial sacs:**
a   Are always accompanied by intestinal obstruction.   (   )

b   Are more common in direct than indirect inguinal herniae.   (   )

c   Are usually irreducible.   (   )
d   Produce local pain and tenderness.   (   )

169 **Incisional herniae are related to:**
a   Wound infections.   (   )
b   Anaemia and malnutrition.   (   )
c   Obesity.   (   )
d   The use of absorbable suture materials.   (   )

170 **Herniae in the umbilical region:**
a   Are always acquired in origin.   (   )

b   Usually occur in males.   (   )
c   Usually require surgical repair in infants.   (   )

d   Rarely strangulate.   (   )

a T− The vast majority of inguinal herniae in childhood are indirect
b T   inguinal herniae within a patent process vaginalis. They do not
c F   obliterate spontaneously and should be treated surgically.
d F− The direct inguinal hernia passes through a diffuse weakness in the
       transversalis fascia and posterior wall of the inguinal canal. It is thus
       most common in old age.

a F− Herniae may produce strangulation of omentum without intestinal
       involvement. Occasionally only part of the intestinal wall is 'threatened'
       (a Richter's hernia) and intestinal obstruction may not occur.
b F− Direct inguinal herniae are less likely to strangulate for they have a wider
       neck and a shorter sac.
c T− Irreducibility is a sign of incarceration of the hernial contents and
d T   strangulation may be imminent. Strangulation produces pain, local
       tenderness and, often, discolouration of the overlying tissues.

a T− These are iatrogenic herniae and the commonest predisposing cause is
b F   an infection of the original surgical wound. There is a greatly increased
c T   incidence in obese patients, possibly because of the increased incidence
d T   of wound haematomata but no definite evidence exists that either
       anaemia or hypoproteinaemia contributes to their formation. The use
       of absorbable suture materials to close aponeurotic sheaths is, possibly,
       a factor in their formation. Catgut loses its tensile strength in 10 to 20
       days and aponeuroses do not gain more than 60 per cent of their
       original strength for 6 to 8 months.

a F− They are of two types: the infantile type which presents at birth is due
       to a congenital weakness in the umbilicus, and the acquired adult type
       which most frequently occurs in obese elderly patients is due to a
       weakness occurring in the linea alba just above the umbilicus. This
       latter type is known as a para-umbilical hernia.
b F− There is not an increased incidence in males.
c F− Those of the infantile type frequently close spontaneously before the
       age of 2 years, especially if the defect is less than 1 cm in diameter.
d F− The para-umbilical hernia is particularly prone to strangulation, and
       surgical repair is thus usually indicated in this group.

171 **A discharge from the umbilicus:**
a May indicate a patent vitello-intestinal duct. ( )

b May indicate an anomaly of the urachus. ( )

c At the time of menstruation may indicate endometriosis. ( )

d In the neonate is of no immediate clinical significance. ( )

172 **An exomphalos:**
a Is a congenital defect of the urethra. ( )
b Is a congenital defect of the anterior abdominal wall. ( )
b Is otherwise known as gastroschisis. ( )

d Needs urgent surgical treatment. ( )

173 **Widespread carcinomatous involvement of the peritoneum:**
a Is frequently confirmed by abdominal paracentesis. ( )

b Can often be diagnosed by rectal examination. ( )

c Indicates that the primary neoplasm is abdominal in origin. ( )

d Is usually associated with jaundice. ( )

a　T— When the vitello-intestinal duct fails to disappear and remains patent throughout its length, a congenital small bowel fistula exists. Other related anomalies include Meckel's diverticulum and a fibrous congenital vitello-intestinal band.

b　T— A patent urachus results in the intermittent discharge of urine from the umbilicus.

c　T— This is rare; the discharge is bloody and arises from ectopic endometrial tissue.

d　F— In addition to the congenital defects already referred to, infection of the umbilicus (omphalitis) in the new born is potentially dangerous because of its rapid spread to the surrounding abdominal wall, peritoneum and, via incompletely obliterated umbilical vessels, to the liver.

a　F— Exomphalos is a herniation of intra-abdominal viscera through the
b　T　umbilical ring. It is covered by a peritoneal sac which often ruptures
c　F　after birth. Gastroschisis is a congenital defect of the abdominal wall and has no membranous covering.

d　T— A proportion of the less severe cases can be treated by primary closure but the majority with an intact sac are treated by dressing with 2 per cent mercurochrome. This allows epithelisation to occur and the ventral hernia can be treated at a later date. A ruptured exomphalos or gastroschisis needs urgent closure. In the larger defects this may be achieved by covering with silastic sheeting which allows epithelisation and staged closure to be undertaken.

a　T— Cytological examination of a sample of ascitic fluid often reveals the presence of exfoliated neoplastic cells.

b　T— The rectovesical or recto-uterine pouch is frequently the site of peritoneal metastatic deposits.

c　F— Disseminated breast cancer frequently results in peritoneal deposits and ascites.

d　F— Although metastases in the liver and porta hepatis are frequently present, there is no close association between peritoneal deposits and jaundice.

174 **Blunt injuries to the abdomen:**
a May cause peritonitis. ( )
b May cause intestinal obstruction. ( )

c May cause acute gastroduodenal ulceration. ( )

d Rarely need urgent laparotomy. ( )

175 **Car seat belts (lap diagonal) when properly adjusted:**
a Prevent injuries to the abdominal viscera. ( )
b May cause small bowel injuries. ( )

c Do not reduce the incidence of head injuries amongst car ( )
passengers involved in a road traffic accident.
d Protect the cervical spine during sudden acceleration. ( )

176 **Indication of a serious intra-abdominal injury in a comatose patient may be gained by:**
a Abdominal paracentesis. ( )
b The observation of pattern bruising on the abdominal wall. ( )

c Falling haemoglobin values. ( )
d The presence of diarrhoea. ( )

177 **Penetrating wounds of the abdomen:**
a Can be adequately explored by a probe. ( )

b Frequently result in acquired abdominal wall herniae. ( )
c May be managed by careful observation, laparotomy being ( )
indicated if signs of peritonitis occur.
d Can be treated conservatively if the weapon is less than 3 cm ( )
long.

a T— Crushing or tearing of the bowel may occur and result in a perforation.
b T   Bleeding from a submucosal vessel may produce an intramural haematoma large enough to cause intestinal obstruction.
c T— 'Stress' ulcers of the stomach and duodenum may follow any hypotensive episode.
d F— The signs of peritonitis, or of intra-abdominal haemorrhage necessitate urgent laparotomy.

a F— Serious injuries to bowel, mesenteric vessels, pancreas and kidney may
b T   still occur during sudden deceleration. It should be emphasised that the injuries would probably have been more serious had a belt not been worn.
c F— Seat belts largely prevent dashboard and windscreen head injuries occurring.
d F— 'Whiplash' injuries to the cervical spine can occur during a sudden acceleration even when seat belts are worn. They may be reduced by the introduction of head rests.

a T— Aspiration of blood or purulent peritoneal fluid suggests visceral injury.
b T— When the pattern of clothing is imprinted on the abdominal wall, it implies that a severe crush injury has occurred.
c T— This may denote a splenic or liver rupture.
d F

a F— The shuttering and overriding actions of the abdominal wall muscles prevent full exploration with a probe.
b F— This is no more common than after laparotomy.
c T— If the patient is observed carefully, an experienced clinician may avoid an unnecessary laparotomy.
d F— Compression of the abdomen wall occurs during penetration, thus al'owing short objects to enter the peritoneal cavity and the viscera.

178 Urinary tract injuries:

a Are usually accompanied by some degree of haematuria. (   )

b Require an urgent intravenous pyelogram and possibly a (   )
cystogram.

c Involving the kidney require urgent surgery. (   )

d Which demonstrate urine extravasating from the bladder are (   )
generally managed conservatively.

179 Injuries to the urethra:

a Are usually confined to the male. (   )
b Are often caused by road traffic accidents. (   )

c Are readily diagnosed on intravenous pyelography. (   )

d Require urgent surgical treatment. (   )

180 Patients with renal trauma:

a Usually present with haematuria. (   )
b Usually require surgical management. (   )

c Always require an intravenous pyelogram. (   )

d Often present with acute renal failure. (   )

181 The spleen:

a Is the commonest organ injured in blunt abdominal trauma. (   )

b Usually continues to bleed once its capsule is torn and its (   )
pulp lacerated.
c Either bleeds immediately or not at all after a pulp injury. (   )
d Should be removed if there has been a laceration of its (   )
capsule.

a   T— The amount of haematuria does not relate to the degree of damage to the urinary tract.

b   T— These two investigations will, in most cases, localise the injury, establish whether the patient has two kidneys and determine the function of each.

c   F— The early management of the injured kidney is, in most cases, by observation.

d   F— Urgent surgery is indicated once this diagnosis is made.

a   F— Fractures of the pelvis in either sex may result in a torn membraneous
b   T   urethra. In the male the prostate and bladder may then be displaced upwards.

c   F— Failure to pass urine, after a pelvic injury, should arouse suspicion and if gentle catheterisation is not possible then urethrograms or laparotomy will be required to establish the diagnosis.

d   T— Diversion of the urinary stream and restoration of urethral continuity should be undertaken in every case in order to avoid extravasation, periurethral fibrosis and stricture formation.

a   T— The commonest results of blunt trauma to the kidney are relatively
b   F   minor contusions or lacerations to the renal parenchyma. These cause loin pain and overt or microscopic haematuria. Surgery is not necessary except in the rare cases of major lacerations or injuries to the renal pedicle.

c   T— This is a most important investigation. Not only may it confirm the suspected injury but it will also present evidence of the presence or absence of the contralateral kidney.

d   F— This is rare but may follow severe injury to a solitary kidney or bilateral severe injuries.

a   T— On account of its thin capsule, proximity to the ribs and its relatively mobile nature.

b   T— A torn capsule with a pulp laceration is unlikely to stop bleeding. A
       pulp laceration lying deep to an intact capsule may produce a sub-
c   F capsular haematoma which develops over a period of days, weeks or
d   T months. Delayed spontaneous haemorrhage will almost certainly ensue.
       It is advisable to remove any spleen which has any signs of trauma.

182   Traumatic rupture of the spleen:

a   Not infrequently presents more than 7 days after the   (   )
causative injury.

b   Frequently presents with shoulder tip pain.   (   )

c   May be diagnosed by paracentesis.   (   )

d   May, in the absence of hypovolaemia, be treated conservatively. (   )

X   The Acute Abdomen

183   Acute abdominal pain which is:

a   Colicky in nature indicates obstruction of a hollow viscus.   (   )

b   Continuous is typical of inflammation.   (   )
c   Maximal in the right loin is typical of duodenal ulceration.   (   )

d   In the right upper quadrant accentuated by inspiration is   (   )
typical of cholecystitis.

184   In the acute abdomen, vomiting:

a   Occurring soon after the onset of colicky pain often   (   )
indicates pathology outside the gastrointestinal tract.

b   Of fluid containing no bile is characteristic of small bowel   (   )
obstruction.
c   Of faeculent fluid usually indicates a gastro-colic fistula.   (   )

d   Is a common early accompaniment of gastroduodenal   (   )
perforation.

a T— In 20 per cent of cases the rupture is delayed for up to 2 weeks after the injury. This is usually due to a delayed rupture of a subcapsular haematoma into the peritoneal cavity.

b T— This is usually left sided and indicates the left sided diaphragmatic irritation that is common in this condition.

c T— A four quadrant paracentesis through a fine needle is valuable in the investigation of any suspected abdominal injury. A negative paracentesis does not exclude the possibility of a haemoperitoneum but a positive aspirate will encourage early laparotomy.

d F— Any suspicion of a ruptured spleen indicates the need for laparotomy. Delayed haemorrhage, when it occurs, is frequently catastrophic.

a T— Ureteric colic arises in the lumbar region and spreads down via the iliac fossa towards the external genitalia; biliary colic will characteristically be maximal in the right upper quadrant; intestinal colic will be referred to the midline anteriorly.

b T— Whether this arises from infection, haemorrhage or ischaemia.

c F— Duodenal pain is felt in the epigastrium. Loin pain is usually of renal origin.

d T— Be aware that diaphragmatic irritation from pleural or pulmonary pathology may produce the same kind of pain.

a T— Both biliary and renal colic produce 'reflex' vomiting coincident with the pain. This will, however, also occur with a high small bowel obstruction.

b F— This almost always indicates gastric pathology, particularly pyloric stenosis.

c F— This is a very rare cause of faeculent vomiting. The usual cause is well developed lower small bowel obstruction. Bacterial proliferation and decomposition of the stagnant bowel contents causes this faeculent change.

d F— Vomiting is an uncommon early symptom in this condition.

185 **Faeculent vomiting:**
a Is commonly seen after upper gastrointestinal tract bleeding. ( )
b Indicates large bowel obstruction. ( )
c Indicates bacterial proliferation in the upper intestinal tract. ( )
d Suggests a gastro-colic fistula. ( )

186 **A patient with generalised peritonitis:**
a Usually has an elevated temperature and pulse rate. ( )
b Characteristically complains of spasmodic severe pain which causes him to be restless. ( )
c Characteristically vomits. ( )
d Will usually have a rapid and deep respiratory pattern. ( )

187 **Perforated duodenal ulcers:**
a Occur most frequently in men. ( )
b Are usually preceded by an exacerbation of ulcer symptoms. ( )
c Are usually accompanied by a leucocytosis. ( )
d Produce abdominal tenderness which is most marked in the epigastrium. ( )

188 **A perforated duodenal ulcer:**
a Usually lies on the anterior or superior surface of the duodenum. ( )
b Usually presents with the acute onset of severe back pain. ( )
c Produces radiological evidence of free gas in the peritoneum in over 90 per cent of the patients. ( )
d Is usually treated by simple closure of the perforation. ( )

a F— Small bowel obstruction always results in bacterial proliferation and decomposition of the small bowel contents then occurs. The smell and
b F   appearance of such vomitus is faeculent. Altered blood is usually
c T   darker and less foul smelling. Faeculent vomiting is a late (and relatively infrequent) sign of large bowel obstruction.
d F— In this rare condition, if vomiting occurs then the vomitus may contain faeces. It does not have the homogeneity of faeculent vomiting.

a T— Though these may take a few hours to develop.
b F— The pain is severe, constant and widespread and the patient lies motionless since movement exacerbates the pain.
c T— This is almost constantly present. At first it is reflex in nature and the volume is small but as the effects of the ensuing paralytic ileus develop the vomit increases in volume.
d F— The respiratory movements though rapid are shallow for diaphragmatic and abdominal wall movements increase the pain.

a T— It is 3 to 4 times more common in males.
b T— The majority of patients have had a recent worsening of ulcer symptoms. A small minority have no previous dyspeptic history.
c T— The leucocyte count usually rises within a few hours due to developing peritonitis.
d T— As in all cases of generalised peritonitis, the abdominal tenderness and rigidity are most marked over the causative lesion.

a T— Penetrating posterior ulcers usually bleed after erosion of the gastro-duodenal artery; anterior ulcers perforate rather than bleed.
b F— By far the commonest presentation is the acute onset of severe epigastric pain which rapidly spreads to the whole abdomen.
c F— Less than 75 per cent of perforated ulcers show free gas under the diaphragm on an erect film of the abdomen.
d T— For acute ulcers and small chronic ulcers this is advised. In perforation of large ulcers definitive surgery, i.e. vagotomy and pyloroplasty or partial gastrectomy is usually preferred providing that peritoneal contamination is neither extensive nor well established.

189 **Congenital pyloric stenosis:**
a   Occurs more commonly in male children.   (   )

b   Usually presents in the first few days of life.   (   )

c   Presents with bile stained vomiting.   (   )

d   Is usually diagnosed on clinical examination.   (   )

190 **Acute appendicitis:**
a   Is most common in the 30 to 40 year age group.   (   )

b   Characteristically presents with a high temperature.   (   )

c   Is often associated with painful extension of the right hip.   (   )

d   May produce haematuria and pyuria.   (   )

191 **Appendicitis is:**
a   More common in females.   (   )
b   Distributed evenly throughout the world's population.   (   )

c   More likely to occur if the appendix is in the retrocaecal   (   )
    position.
d   Commonly the result of appendicular obstruction.   (   )

a   T—   Boys are affected four times as commonly as girls. There is some evidence of a hereditary tendency.

b   F—   The signs of pyloric obstruction usually present after the second week of life. By this time oedema of the pyloric mucosa contributes to the narrowing produced by the hypertrophied pyloric muscle to cause obstruction.

c   F—   Projectile vomiting, particularly after feeds, occurs, but this is not bile stained since the obstruction is proximal to the ampulla of Vater.

d   T—   If the abdomen is examined after the infant has been fed, forceful transverse peristaltic waves can usually be seen passing from left to right across the upper abdomen and the abnormal mass of hypertrophied muscle, the 'pyloric tumour', becomes palpable. Surgical treatment is indicated once fluid and electrolyte imbalance has been corrected.

a   F—   The peak incidence is in the 15 to 25 year age group. It is uncommon in the very young and the very old (but more dangerous and difficult to diagnose).

b   F—   Temperature and pulse are frequently normal early in the disease. The temperature rarely exceeds 38°C unless perforation or abscess formation has occurred.

c   T—   The retrocaecal position is the most common and in this position the inflamed appendix may produce spasm of iliopsoas and painful limited extension of the right hip. This is a useful diagnostic sign.

d   T—   Right sided renal and ureteric colic are frequently confused with appendicitis. The detection of red cells in the urine usually indicates urinary calculi as the cause. However an inflamed appendix that lies adjacent to the right ureter or bladder may produce urinary symptoms such as haematuria and pyuria.

a   F—   The incidence is the same in both sexes.

b   F—   The disease is uncommon in the underdeveloped countries of the Third World.

c   F—   Though this is the commonest position of the appendix, it carries no increased risk of appendicitis.

d   T—   Appendicitis follows obstruction of the appendicular lumen due either to lymphoid hyperplasia (which is particularly common in children), a faecolith (which is found in almost half the cases) or, rarely, to a tumour or stricture.

192 **The physical signs of early appendicitis:**
a Are generally of more diagnostic value than the patient's ( )
history.
b Usually include muscle guarding in the right iliac fossa. ( )

c Usually include a pyrexia above 38.5°C. ( )

d Do not include rectal tenderness. ( )

193 **Patients with early appendicitis:**
a Usually present with central abdominal pain. ( )

b Rarely present with anorexia. ( )
c Have usually vomited on one or two occasions. ( )
d Usually complain of similar attacks of pain in the previous ( )
few weeks.

194 **Investigation of a case of acute appendicitis:**
a Will usually reveal a polymorphonuclear leucocytosis. ( )
b Often shows microscopic haematuria. ( )
c Usually reveals haemoconcentration. ( )

d Often reveals fluid levels in the right iliac fossa on an erect ( )
X-ray of the abdomen.

195 **Likely differential diagnoses in a young woman with**
appendicitis include:
a Ovulatory pain. ( )
b Ruptured ectopic pregnancy. ( )

c Colonic diverticulitis. ( )
d Caecal carcinoma. ( )

a F— Usually the reverse is true.

b T— This resistance to palpation is a guide to the severity of the inflammation and it progresses to involuntary rigidity.

c F— A milder pyrexia is common. High fever is uncommon until perforation or abscess formation occurs.

d F— A rectal examination should always be performed. Rectal tenderness in the pouch of Douglas may provide the only positive evidence of appendicitis when the inflamed organ lies in the pelvis.

a T— This is felt most severely in the umbilical region. In a few cases such a history is not obtained.

b F— Anorexia is almost always noted in patients with appendicitis.

c T— This follows the abdominal pain and may be reflex in nature.

d F— Though recurrent appendicitis occasionally occurs it is rare. A history of previous abdominal pain should alert the clinician to think of other causes of the abdominal pain.

a T— Too much emphasis should not be placed on laboratory tests for their

b T   discriminatory value is slight. Though there is usually a leucocytosis

c F   this is not constant. About one quarter of patients will show leucocytes or red cells in the urine but there is rarely a raised haematocrit in the early case.

d F— Abdominal radiology is not often helpful. When there is radiological evidence of appendicitis (such as the absence of small bowel gas in the right iliac fossa, gas under the diaphragm or a scoliosis concave to the right), the diagnosis is usually clinically obvious.

a T— Midcycle ovulatory pain lasts for only a few hours.

b T— Often there is a history of a missed menstruation and the presence of a tender tubal mass is noted on pelvic examination.

c F— Colonic diverticulitis and caecal cancer may mimic appendicitis, but it is

d F   extremely uncommon for these to occur in this age group.

196 **Appendicectomy should be undertaken:**
a   After laparotomy reveals a diagnosis of mesenteric adenitis.   (   )

b   Immediately in adult patients with an appendix abscess.   (   )

c   In patients with a gangrenous appendix.   (   )
d   In patients with chronic appendicitis.   (   )

197 **Obstruction of the lumen of the appendix may lead to:**
a   Mucosal ulceration.   (   )
b   Gangrenous appendicitis.   (   )
c   A perforated appendix.   (   )

d   Intussusception of the appendix.   (   )

198 **In the differential diagnosis of appendicitis in an infant it is important to consider:**
a   Ileo-ileal intussusception.   (   )

b   Basal pneumonia.   (   )
c   Henoch-Schoenlein purpura.   (   )

d   Torsion of an ovarian cyst.   (   )

199 **Acute non-specific mesenteric lymphadenitis:**
a   Is commonest between 5 and 12 years of age.   (   )
b   Is usually associated with an upper respiratory tract infection.   (   )

c   Is usually associated with cervical lymphadenopathy.   (   )

d   Is characterised by enlarged mesenteric lymph nodes which are infected by gram-negative organisms.   (   )

a   T— The procedure is prophylactic and carries little additional morbidity and mortality.

b   F— It is usually wisest to surgically drain the abscess and unless the appendix can be removed easily it should be left for an interval appendicectomy some 2 months later.

c   T— In all cases.

d   T— This disputed condition occurs but is not common.

a   T— Luminal obstruction leads to oedema and distension of the distal

b   T   appendix, mucosal ulcers appear and as the distension increases the

c   T   venous drainage and arterial supply are impeded and gangrenous perforation may occur. Peritonitis may then follow and the mortality rises.

d   F— This is not related.

a   T— Screaming and intermittent abdominal colic, a short history of melaena and palpation of a sausage-shaped mass may indicate an intussusception.

b   T— Diaphragmatic pleurisy may produce referred pain in the lower abdomen.

c   T— A haematoma of the small bowel wall may mimic appendicitis but the presence of a purpuric rash and joint pains should arouse suspicion of Henoch-Schoenlein purpura.

d   F— This is very uncommon before puberty.

a   T— Although it is less common than appendicitis in this age group.

b   T— This is commonly coexistent with, or precedes the vague, colicky, lower abdominal pain by a few days.

c   T— There is frequently pharyngeal injection. Examination of the abdomen reveals tenderness which is higher, more medial and more variable in position than appendicitis. The leucocyte count is moderately raised to 12 000 to 15 000/mm^3. (12 000 to 15 000/μl).

d   F— Although mesenteric lymph node enlargement is characteristically present, cultures of the nodes are usually sterile.

200 **Abdominal distension in mechanical intestinal obstruction is produced in part by:**

a   Swallowed air.   (   )

b   Carbon dioxide produced in the bowel.   (   )

c   Increased intestinal secretions proximal to the obstruction.   (   )
d   Decreased intestinal absorption proximal to the obstruction.   (   )

201 **The level of intestinal obstruction can be determined by:**

a   Questioning the patient.   (   )

b   Examining the patient.   (   )

c   Radiological examination of the patient.   (   )

d   Repeated measurements of the patient's girth.   (   )

202 **Acute small bowel obstruction:**

a   Is commonly caused by postoperative adhesions.   (   )

b   Accompanied by the signs of peritonitis, suggests bowel strangulation. (   )

c   Is often associated with a raised serum amylase.   (   )

d   Generally produces abdominal distension within 2 to 3 hours of onset. (   )

a T— Nitrogen is not readily absorbed by the intestine, thus more than 70 per cent of the accumulated gas comes from swallowed air.
b F— Though large quantities of carbon dioxide are produced in the bowel, accumulation does not occur because this gas is readily absorbed.
c T— In the distended bowel there is a gross disturbance of the usual
d T   absorption/secretion activities of the intestinal mucosa. Both increased secretion and decreased absorption of fluid have been shown to occur in a distended bowel proximal to an obstruction.

a T— In high small bowel obstruction vomiting occurs soon after the onset of pain whereas in large bowel obstruction vomiting appears much later if at all. Small bowel colic is felt in the central abdomen; large bowel colic in the suprapubic region. Constipation is an early symptom in large bowel obstruction.
b T— In large bowel obstruction distension is greater and tends to be most marked in the flanks. The distension of small bowel obstruction is central abdominal.
c T— In small bowel obstruction there is very little gas in the colon. Colonic distension can usually be distinguished from small bowel distension by haustral markings which occupy only part of the transverse diameter of the bowel. In distended small bowel, mucosal folds, the valvulae conniventes, can be seen traversing the whole diameter.
d F— Except in high small bowel obstruction progressive increase in the patient's abdominal girth is a feature of all types of intestinal obstruction.

a T— Adhesions and external herniae are the two commonest causes. A careful inspection for surgical scars and of the hernial orifices must therefore be routine.
b T— A rising temperature and pulse rate and local abdominal tenderness and rigidity, all indicate that strangulation is developing. Operative treatment is then an urgent necessity.
c T— The serum amylase is frequently raised to twice normal values but should not be confused with the very high values usually seen in the initial stages of acute pancreatitis.
d F— Central abdominal distension usually appears after 12 to 24 hours and may be absent in high small bowel obstruction.

203 **In the treatment of intestinal obstruction:**

a Nasogastric suction should be instituted preoperatively. ( )

b Intravenous fluid replacement is essential. ( )

c Immediate surgery is essential. ( )

d Surgery should be restricted to those cases where strangula- ( )
lation is diagnosed.

204 **Emergency treatment of a mechanical obstruction of the**
large bowel may include:

a Enemata. ( )

b Exteriorisation and resection of the lesion. ( )
c A transverse colostomy. ( )
d An ileo-transverse colostomy. ( )

205 **Strangulation of the bowel:**

a Commonly complicates closed loop obstruction. ( )

b Is difficult to distinguish from simple intestinal obstruction. ( )

c Is accompanied by bleeding into the affected bowel. ( )

d Frequently causes peritonitis. ( )

a T— Aspiration via a nasogastric tube, though having little effect on the distended bowel, minimises further distension by removing swallowed air. It also reduces the risk of aspiration of vomit. All patients with intestinal

b T   obstruction will have abnormal fluid and electrolyte losses—these must be made good by the intravenous administration of isotonic saline, often with potassium supplements.

c F— Although in many cases the most appropriate treatment is surgical relief of the obstruction, this should not be performed until careful attention has been paid to correcting fluid and electrolyte deficiencies and nasogastric suction has been instituted.

d F— Strangulation is a serious complication adding peritonitis to the pathophysiology of intestinal obstruction. This is reflected in a high mortality rate of more than 25 per cent, and therefore surgery is preferable before this complication develops.

a T— Faecal impaction is a cause of large bowel obstruction in the elderly. It may be effectively treated by enemata though disimpaction under general anaesthetic is frequently necessary.

b T— Each of these procedures may have some part to play. It is usually unsafe

c T   to attempt resection of the obstructing lesion with primary anastomosis

d T   and the majority of cases are managed in the first instance by these simpler methods which permit safe decompression of the proximal bowel.

a T— When the bowel lumen is closed at two points along its length the raised intraluminal pressure results in impairment of the blood supply to the affected loop and strangulation frequently occurs.

b F— Strangulation should be suspected in any patient with intestinal obstruction who demonstrates signs of local or generalised peritonitis.

c T— Blood and plasma are lost from the strangulated portion and trapped in it following venous obstruction and capillary leakage. As an approximate guide, one litre of blood may be lost per metre of strangulated bowel.

d T— The ischaemic segment of bowel is permeable to the increased numbers of bacteria and their toxins. This toxic fluid produces peritonitis and its absorption into the general circulation can cause cardiovascular collapse.

206 **Small bowel obstruction often results in:**
a Hyperkalaemia.   (   )
b Metabolic alkalosis.   (   )

c Oliguria.   (   )
d Hypovolaemia.   (   )

207 **Large bowel obstruction:**
a Is most commonly caused by diverticular disease of the   (   )
colon.

b Has its maximum incidence before the age of 50.   (   )
c Frequently presents with nausea and vomiting.   (   )

d Usually heralds its onset with constant suprapubic pain.   (   )

208 **Patients with acute colonic diverticulitis:**
a Often give a history of recent lower abdominal colic.   (   )

b Often present with a pyrexia.   (   )

c Can be frequently diagnosed on sigmoidoscopic appearances.   (   )

d Frequently develop faecal peritonitis.   (   )

209 **Acute pancreatitis typically:**
a Is accompanied by hypercalcaemia.   (   )

b Produces paralytic ileus.   (   )

c Is associated with a pleural effusion.   (   )

d Produces pyloric stenosis.   (   )

a   F— Potassium is lost in intestinal secretions, in vomiting and in abnormal
b   T   renal losses which follow attempts to conserve hydrogen ions in the
         metabolic alkalosis that accompanies proximal small bowel obstruction.
c   T— Dehydration rapidly develops due to loss of fluid into the distended
d   T   bowel, diminished fluid intake and vomiting. Haemoconcentration,
         hypovolaemia and oliguria thus rapidly appear.

a   F— Colonic cancer is the most common cause, followed by diverticular
         disease and sigmoid volvulus. Most of the obstructing cancers are in the
         descending and sigmoid colon.
b   F— This is a disease of the elderly.
c   F— These symptoms are usually absent until the late stages of the disease,
         particularly when the ileocaecal valve is competent.
d   F— The visceral pain produced is vague but colicky and felt in the lower
         abdomen.

a   T— These symptoms of diverticular disease frequently precede the acute
         attack.
b   T— Temperatures of 38°C and above may indicate the presence of a
         pericolic abscess.
c   F— Though oedema of the rectosigmoid junction may occasionally be seen,
         the more inaccessible pelvic colon is the site of the pathology, and out
         of reach of the sigmoidoscope.
d   F— Rupture of a pericolic abscess may lead to generalised peritonitis. This
         complication, which carries a high mortality, is rare. The inflammation
         more frequently localises as a pericolic abscess.

a   F— Hypocalcaemia is a frequent complication occurring within a few days of
         the onset. Though it is frequently stated to be a consequence of
         saponification of retroperitoneal fat, this is almost certainly a too
         facile explanation and the true cause is still unknown.
b   T— Even mild attacks generally produce a segmental ileus of the overlying
         jejunal loops. The distended bowel in the upper abdomen produces
         characteristic radiological appearances.
c   T— Most commonly a left sided effusion, due to subdiaphragmatic
         inflammation.
d   F— However there is frequently distortion of the duodenal loop on a barium
         meal.

210   Acute pancreatitis:

a   Often simulates a perforated peptic ulcer in its presentation.   (   )

b   Often presents with the signs of hypovolaemia.   (   )

c   Can readily be distinguished from other causes of acute abdominal pain by the presence of a raised serum amylase.   (   )

d   Frequently has a raised concentration of urinary amylase.   (   )

211   The treatment of acute pancreatitis:

a   Is largely nonspecific and supportive.   (   )

b   Should include a laparotomy in the majority of cases.   (   )

c   Should routinely include the administration of calcium.   (   )

d   Should routinely include the administration of antibiotics.   (   )

212   Childhood intussusception:

a   Usually presents during the first year of life.   (   )

b   Is frequently ileocolic.   (   )

c   Can usually be diagnosed without X-ray examination of the abdomen.   (   )

d   Rarely requires surgical treatment.   (   )

a   T— The disease varies in severity and the epigastric pain may be as severe as that of a perforated peptic ulcer. It commonly radiates to the back and then must be distinguished from a ruptured or dissecting aortic aneurysm.

b   T— In a severe attack there is considerable retroperitoneal inflammation and sequestration of fluid which results in hypovolaemia and shock.

c   F— Although in most cases the serum amylase rises within 8 hours of the onset and remains elevated for 2 to 3 days only a rise of approximately

d   T   four times the normal value will certainly distinguish pancreatitis from the other causes of hyperamylasaemia, viz. gallstones, perforated peptic ulcer, small bowel obstruction and mesenteric thrombosis. There is a more constant rise in urinary amylase values in pancreatitis than in the above conditions.

a   T— Hypovolaemia should be corrected, continuous nasogastric suction will relieve distension and reduce pancreatic secretion while pain relief can usually be achieved with pethidine.

b   F— Most cases will improve on the above therapy but laparotomy is advised if the patient is deteriorating or if a fever or abdominal mass appears. Usually removal of the necrotic tissue and drainage of the area is all that can be undertaken.

c   F— It should only be given in those patients who have clinical or biochemical evidence of hypocalcaemia.

d   F— Antibiotics are essential in the treatment of any infective complications but their prophylactic use is debatable.

a   T— The average age of presentation is gradually becoming younger. The cause

b   T   is obscure. It is suggested lymphatic hyperplasia secondary to virus infections or a change in the infant's diet on weaning, may produce a submucosal swelling in the intestinal wall which initiates the intussusception.

c   T— Sudden colicky pain, often with the passage of bloody stools, suggests the diagnosis—the palpation of a sausage-shaped mass in the right upper quadrant is confirmatory.

d   F— Providing no signs of intestinal strangulation exist then *gentle* reduction by means of a barium enema may be attempted under fluoroscopic control. The majority of patients, however, require surgical intervention.

213   Meconium ileus:

a   Is the presenting feature in the majority of patients with   (   )
     cystic fibrosis.

b   Is associated with achlorhydria.   (   )

c   Presents with a distended abdomen and bilious vomiting.   (   )

d   May be effectively treated with acetyl cysteine.   (   )

214   Neonatal duodenal obstruction:

a   May be associated with Down's syndrome.   (   )

b   Is more frequently found in premature infants.   (   )

c   Typically presents with gross abdominal distension.   (   )

d   Usually presents with vomiting of bile stained fluid.   (   )

215   Acute superior mesenteric artery occlusion:

a   Characteristically presents with sudden pain and tenderness   (   )
     of increasing intensity.

b   Is frequently accompanied by overt or occult blood loss in   (   )
     the stools.

c   Frequently produces peritonitis.   (   )

d   Can usually be diagnosed on plain abdominal X-rays.   (   )

216   A ruptured ectopic pregnancy:

a   Usually occurs in the first month of pregnancy.   (   )

b   Usually presents with severe lower abdominal pain.   (   )

c   Frequently presents with hypovolaemic shock.   (   )

d   Can usually be diagnosed by pelvic examination.   (   )

a F— Only about 10 per cent of patients with cystic fibrosis have meconium ileus.
b F— No abnormalities of gastric secretion occur in this syndrome. There is an associated deficiency of pancreatic function.
c T— Distal ileal obstruction occurs due to abnormally viscous meconium.
d T   This obstruction must usually be relieved surgically or, in mild cases, by the detergent action of orally administered acetyl cysteine or gastrografin, a hypertonic contrast medium.

a T— More than 20 per cent of such infants will also have Down's syndrome.
b F— There is not an increased frequency in premature infants.
c F— The obstruction is high and so abdominal distension is usually absent.
d T— Vomiting is frequent, and usually contains bile since the obstruction is usually distal to the ampulla of Vater.

a T— The pain is often more severe than the abdominal tenderness suggests.
b T— Intestinal blood loss is almost invariably present and results from haemorrhagic infarction of the bowel mucosa.
c T— Ischaemia of the bowel leads to the bacteria of the bowel 'leaking' into the peritoneal cavity with catastrophic results.
d F— X-rays are usually unhelpful. Occasionally intra-hepatic gas is seen as the ominous result of gas forming organisms ascending via the portal vein to the liver.

a F— Rupture usually occurs between the sixth and twelfth weeks of pregnancy. There is often a history of a missed or scanty menstrual period.
b T— This is associated with vomiting and a desire to defaecate.
c T— A large proportion of patients with this life-threatening condition suffer a rapid and severe blood loss.
d T— A tender cervix and a boggy mass in the vaginal fornices are usually palpable.

217 Biliary colic typically:
  a Occurs 3 to 4 hours after meals.   (   )
  b Lasts 5 to 20 minutes.   (   )
  .c Radiates from the upper abdomen to the right subscapular   (   )
     region.
  d Is made worse by deep inspiration.   (   )

XI Stomach, Duodenum and Small Intestine

218 Benign gastric ulcers:
  a Occur in the same age group as duodenal ulcers.   (   )

  b Are more common in males than females.   (   )
  c Are more common in the upper social classes.   (   )
  d Produce epigastric pain after eating food.   (   )

219 Uncomplicated benign gastric ulcers:
  a Occur most commonly on the greater curve of the stomach.   (   )

  b Should initially be treated medically.   (   )

  c Commonly recur after medical treatment.   (   )

  d Should receive surgical treatment if healing has not occurred   (   )
     after 4 to 6 weeks of medical.

a   F—   The patient usually gives a past history of dyspepsia, viz. postprandial
b   F   flatulence, nausea and epigastric pain. Biliary colic usually occurs soon
c   T   after a meal and lasts at least 3 to 4 hours and often a day or more.
         The pain is initially felt in the epigastrium or right hypochondrium and
d   T   later radiates to the back or right subscapular region. It is accentuated by
         deep breathing.

a   F—   They are commoner in older people. The peak incidence for duodenal
         ulcers is around 30 years whereas gastric ulcers are most common around
         50 years of age.
b   T—   The disease is twice as common in men.
c   F—   There is an increased incidence in the lower social classes.
d   T—   The pain of gastric ulceration is characteristically felt in the epigastrium
         and is made worse by eating or drinking strong alcoholic beverages.

a   F—   The commonest site is on the lesser curve, particularly around the
         incisura angularis.
b   T—   Particularly if gastroscopy and endoscopic biopsy indicate that the ulcer
         is benign.
c   T—   Recurrence rates of as high as 50 per cent have been reported after
         intensive medical management with antacids, carbenoxolone and bed
         rest.
d   T—   If gastroscopic or X-ray evidence of healing has not occurred at the end of
         this period then surgical treatment (usually a Billroth 1 partial
         gastrectomy with excision of the ulcer) should be undertaken. These
         patients are at risk from haemorrhage or perforation. Awareness of the
         fact that approximately 5 per cent of indolent non-healing benign ulcers
         may be ulcerating cancers masquerading in a benign guise gives further
         justification to this 'aggressive' approach to treatment.

220 Gastric cancer:
a Is more common in males than females. ( )

b Is more common in the higher social classes. ( )

c Is increasing in frequency in the United Kingdom. ( )

d Is more common in rural areas. ( )

221 There is an association of gastric cancer with:
a Achlorhydria of the stomach. ( )

b Atrophic gastritis. ( )

c Adenomatous gastric polyps. ( )

d Duodenal ulceration. ( )

222 Surgical treatment of gastric cancer:
a Should preferably be by a total gastrectomy. ( )

b Gives overall 5 year survival figures of 5 to 10 per cent. ( )

c Includes excision of the tumour as a palliative measure. ( )

d Should be advised for all diagnosed cases. ( )

a T— Throughout the world the incidence in males is approximately twice that of females.

b F— Studies from Scandinavia, Japan, U.S.A. and the U.K. all indicate an increased incidence in the lower social classes.

c F— The incidence is decreasing slightly in the U.K. as in most western countries. This is most striking in the U.S.A. where incidence rates in the 1960s were one third those in the 1930s.

d F— Most epidemiological work has shown an increased incidence in urban areas.

a T— A three- to four-fold increase in incidence has frequently been observed in achlorhydric patients with pernicious anaemia. The majority of patients with gastric cancer have achlorhydria or hypochlorhydria.

b T— Long term follow-up of patients with atrophic gastritis has revealed that a higher than expected incidence of gastric cancer is present.

c T— Gastric polyps are rare but approximately 20 per cent of them are malignant, especially those which are greater than 2 cm in diameter.

d F— There is no association. Indeed gastric cancer is extremely uncommon in patients with active duodenal ulceration.

a F— The development of more radical surgical methods to treat stomach cancer has not improved the survival figures except in the case of carcinomas of the cardia.

b T— Surgical series do report higher 5 year survival in those patients having gastrectomies but the resectability rate is rarely higher than 70 per cent. The 5 year survival rate for patients who had no lymph node metastases at the time of operation is over 40 per cent.

c T— Excision is usually more effective palliation than bypass procedures though the mortality is slightly higher.

d F— At least 20 per cent of the patients will present with signs of incurable disease such as a malignant liver enlargement, malignant ascites or a palpable left supraclavicular node. Only necessary palliation should be attempted in these cases.

223 **The signs and symptoms of potentially curable gastric cancer:**
a May simulate those of a benign gastric ulcer.   (   )

b Include a hard palpable left supraclavicular node.   (   )

c Require investigation by a barium meal examination.   (   )
d Require investigation by a gastroscopic examination even   (   )
   when the barium meal is normal.

224 **Gastric cancer:**
a Is most common in the fundus of the stomach.   (   )

b Is most commonly a squamous cell carcinoma.   (   )
c Frequently metastasises via the blood stream.   (   )

d Is most frequently an ulcerating lesion.   (   )

225 **Treatment of symptomatic duodenal ulcers:**
a Should include twice daily antacids.   (   )

b Should include a strict dietary regime of bland foodstuffs.   (   )

c Should include anti-cholinergic drugs.   (   )

d Should be by early surgery.   (   )

a T— Pain is the commonest first symptom and may mimic that of gastric or
        duodenal ulceration. It thus demands a full investigation when appearing
        in any patient over the age of 50.
b F— Neoplastic involvement of Virchow's node is a sign of widespread
        incurable malignancy originating in the upper gastrointestinal tract.
c T— The diagnostic accuracy of a barium meal for stomach cancer is
d T   approximately 80 per cent. For this reason a negative barium meal in a
        patient suspected of stomach cancer should be followed by a gastroscopic
        examination.

a F— Most cancers are situated around the prepyloric and antral regions,
        especially along the lesser curve.
b F— Almost all the carcinomas are adenocarcinomas.
c T— It spreads via the portal blood to produce liver metastases. Systemic
        blood spread is less common. In addition it may spread by lymphatic
        permeation, direct extension to neighbouring structures and
        transcoelomically to produce peritoneal and ovarian metastases.
d F— Ulcerating cancers form the minority. The majority have a polypoid
        form or are diffusely infiltrating (linitis plastica).

a F— Antacids achieve symptomatic relief by increasing the intragastric pH.
        However, as this effect does not last longer than 1 hour frequent
        administration is necessary.
b F— Some patients recognise foods that cause exacerbations of pain and avoid
        those foods. However, in general, dietary control has no part to play in
        the management of these ulcers.
c F— To be effective in reducing acid output these drugs must be given in
        doses large enough to be associated with a high incidence of unpleasant
        side effects. For this reason they are not generally recommended.
d F— Duodenal ulcers are extremely common but of very varying severity.
        Many symptoms are short lived and of minor consequence. The usual
        indications for surgery are severe and protracted discomfort or
        complications.

226 **Duodenal ulcers:**
a Have an equal incidence in both sexes. ( )
b Have a clinical course characterised by long periods of ( )
remission.
c Are characterised by postprandial pain. ( )

d Occur most commonly in the duodenal cap. ( )

227 **Acute haemorrhage from a duodenal ulcer:**
a Requires an urgent barium meal examination. ( )
b Requires an urgent gastroscopy. ( )

c Should be treated surgically as soon as the diagnosis is made. ( )

d Indicates the presence of a chronic duodenal ulcer. ( )

228 **Post-gastrectomy nutritional disturbances may result in:**
a Megaloblastic anaemia. ( )

b Steatorrhoea. ( )

c Iron deficiency anaemia. ( )

d Osteoporosis. ( )

229 **The incidence of Crohn's disease:**
a Is distributed evenly throughout the world's population. ( )

b Is similar in the two sexes. ( )
c Is highest amongst young adults. ( )
d Is increased in the close relatives of patients with the disease. ( )

124

a   F—   They are 4 to 5 times more common in males.

b   T—   This 'periodicity' of the symptoms, wherein remissions alternate with exacerbations lasting from one week to many months, is characteristic.

c   F—   The epigastric pain generally appears several hours after eating, and thus quite commonly awakes the patient from sleep. It is frequently relieved by food.

d   T—   95 per cent of ulcers are in the first 1.5 cm of the duodenum (the duodenal cap).

a   T—   Diagnosis of the source of the haemorrhage should be sought urgently

b   T   in order that rational treatment may be instituted. These two investigations are complementary in achieving this aim.

c   F—   The majority of haemorrhages from duodenal ulcers do not require urgent surgery. Surgery is indicated when the estimated blood loss is more than 1.5 litres, or when there is a second major haemorrhage within a few days of the first. Since old poeple stand hypovolaemia poorly surgery should be undertaken at an earlier stage in this group.

d   F—   Acute duodenal ulcers frequently bleed and this is particularly common in those associated with major burn injury (Curling's ulcer) or multiple injuries.

a   T—   Megaloblastic anaemia results either from the loss of intrinsic factor following excision of the parietal cells or vitamin B_{12} deficiency caused by bacterial growth in the blind duodenal loop.

b   T—   This probably results from rapid gastric emptying or the food bypassing the duodenum and failing to mix with the bile salts in those patients with a gastrojejunal anastomosis.

c   T—   Iron deficiency is mainly the result of hypochlorhydria and diminished iron absorption.

d   T—   This occurs in about 5 per cent of patients, 10 years after partial gastrectomy. The reasons are obscure.

a   F—   It is almost unknown in the tropics. Its incidence is highest in the Northern latitudes.

b   T—   This is apparent at all ages.

c   T—   The mean age of onset is 25 years, but no age is exempt.

d   T—   Between 2 and 6 per cent of cases have been found in the family of patients with the disease.

230 **Crohn's disease:**
a Has an infective aetiology. ( )
b Is limited to the bowel mucosa. ( )
c Does not produce mucosal ulceration. ( )
d Is characterised by the absence of fibrous tissue in the ( )
affected inflamed bowel.

231 **Patients with Crohn's disease characteristically present with:**
a Colicky abdominal pain. ( )

b Constipation. ( )

c Nutritional deficiencies. ( )

d Rectal bleeding. ( )

232 **In the treatment of patients with Crohn's disease:**
a Medical methods have no part to play. ( )

b Surgery should be the primary method of treatment. ( )

c Steroids may provide a remission in the progress of the disease. ( )

d A high bulk diet should be considered. ( )

a F— Repeated attempts to identify any infective agent have failed.
b F— Lymphoedema is almost always present in the affected bowel and
c F   mesentery—this is associated with a granulomatous inflammatory process
d F   spreading through the whole thickness of the bowel wall. The mucosal
        surface becomes oedematous and interrupted by longitudinal ulcers
        producing the typical 'cobblestone' appearance. There is always extensive
        fibrosis associated with the inflammatory process. This results in the
        frequent development of stenotic bowel lesions.

a T— This is the commonest symptom and is related to the increased motility
        proximal to a partially obstructed bowel.
b F— Diarrhoea is almost always present, being the result of partial obstruction,
        impaired absorption of fluid and bile salts by the diseased bowel,
        bacterial proliferation in a stagnant loop or any combination of these
        factors.
c T— Bacterial proliferation in stagnant loops of small bowel impairs food
        absorption, leads to multiple vitamin deficiencies, macrocytic anaemia
        and steatorrhoea. Loss of weight also results from the anorexia which
        marks the acute disease.
d F— Occult blood loss is almost always present and though anal fissures and
        fistulae are frequently present overt rectal bleeding is rare.

a F— Though no drug at present is known to permanently alter the course of
        the disease, a great improvement can be achieved by supportive
        measures, e.g. codeine and diphenoxylate will improve the diarrhoea and
        abdominal cramps; cholestyramine may reduce the faecal water loss by
        binding bile salts; steatorrhoea may be improved by a low fat diet and
        antibiotics which deal with the bacteria of a stagnant loop; iron, vitamin
        B_{12} and folate may be required to deal with anaemia and the use of an
        'elemental diet' or parenteral hyperalimentation may improve the patient's
        nutrition.
b F— Though surgery has a large part to play, it is only indicated to deal with
        the complications such as intestinal obstruction, inflammatory masses or
        abscesses in the abdomen, internal or external bowel fistulae and indolent
        anal lesions. Surgery should not be undertaken in the absence of these
        complications.
c T— Steroids will induce a remission in the majority of patients and thus have
        a role in management of the acute case. Prolonged use, however, does
        not confer further benefit to the patient.
d F— This is likely to accentuate those symptoms produced by stenotic bowel
        lesions.

233 **Tumours of the small bowel:**
a Are rare. ( )
b May be an inherited disorder. ( )

c Most commonly present with overt or occult rectal bleeding. ( )

d Most commonly present in childhood. ( )

234 **Carcinoid tumours of the gastrointestinal tract:**
a Are most commonly located in the appendix. ( )

b Are usually malignant. ( )

c Arise in the submucosa. ( )

d Are frequently the cause of gastrointestinal haemorrhage. ( )

235 **The carcinoid syndrome:**
a Characteristically includes abdominal cramps. ( )

b Is produced by the release of vasoconstricting substances from the tumour. ( )

c Occurs most commonly with metastatic carcinoid tumours. ( )

d Is usually cured by excision of the primary tumour. ( )

236 **Chronic radiation injury to the intestinal tract:**
a Typically presents with mucosal atrophy. ( )

b Often presents with perforation of the bowel. ( )

c Frequently presents with intestinal obstruction. ( )

d May present with malabsorption. ( )

a   T— They only account for 1 to 2 per cent of all gastrointestinal tumours.
b   T— Intestinal polyposis with melanin pigmentation of the lips, oral mucosa,
and palmar and plantar skin is inherited as a Mendelian dominant
(Peutz-Jeghers syndrome).
c   F— Intestinal obstruction is more common. This is caused by an intussusception or by the annular intramural spread of a malignant tumour.
d   F— The majority of patients present after the age of 45 years.

a   T— Whilst they have been found throughout the gastrointestinal tract, the
appendix is the commonest site, followed by the small intestine.
Bronchial, ovarian and bladder carcinoids also occur.
b   F— The majority are benign, particularly those of the appendix. About 30
per cent of small bowel carcinoids do metastasise.
c   T— They arise from granular cells in the crypts of Lieberkühn and usually
grow submucosally.
d   F— Mucosal ulceration is uncommon, thus bleeding is rare. A more common
complication is intestinal obstruction. Appendiceal carcinoids may
initiate luminal obstruction and cause appendicitis.

a   T— These occur together with flushing over the upper half of the body,
diarrhoea, wheezing and dyspnoea. The symptoms are often precipitated
by food.
b   F— Vasodilator substances, serotonin, β-hydroxyindoleacetic acid, kallikrein
and histamine are released by the tumour.
c   T— The appearance of the syndrome nearly always indicates hepatic
d   F   metastases. Although primary carcinoids produce the vasodilator
substances, systemic effects are uncommon for they are inactivated on
their passage through the liver.

a   F— The injury produces a progressive vasculitis and an associated fibrosis.
Epithelial damage, if it occurs, is probably due to the resultant tissue
hypoxia.
b   T— The impaired blood supply and progressive fibrosis result in the
c   T   intestine becoming thick walled and stenotic with loops bound to each
d   T   other by fibrous adhesions. Ulceration and perforation of the bowel may
occur. Partial or complete obstruction is common and malabsorption
may result from the stagnation of the bowel contents.

237 **Acute radiation injury to the intestinal tract:**
a Commonly presents with intestinal perforation. ( )
b Characteristically produces sloughing of the intestinal ( )
mucosa.
c Is rarely seen when therapeutic doses of radiation are given ( )
to the abdomen and pelvis.

d Is not seen when the patient is exposed to less than 400 rads. ( )

238 **The 'blind-loop' syndrome often:**
a Presents with signs of malnutrition. ( )

b Presents as a complication of Crohn's disease. ( )

c Responds to treatment with oral penicillin. ( )

d Shows a reduced excretion of vitamin B_{12} after an ( )
intramuscular injection of the vitamin.

239 **A Meckel's diverticulum of the small intestine:**
a Is situated at the jejuno-ileal junction. ( )

b Contains all coats of intestinal wall. ( )
c May be associated with a fibrous band connecting it to ( )
the umbilicus.

d Most commonly presents as diverticulitis. ( )

a F— The most vulnerable cells are those of the mucous membranes and high
b T   doses will result in sloughing of the mucosa, haemorrhage and diarrhoea.
       Perforation does not occur in the acute stage but may occur later.
c F— Nausea, vomiting, intestinal cramps and diarrhoea are common when the
       pelvis is irradiated for carcinoma of the cervix or when the abdomen is
       irradiated in the treatment of testicular tumours. These effects subside
       after cessation of therapy and generally require only symptomatic relief.
d F— The effects of irradiation are related to the size of the field to which the
       body is exposed. 400 rads is the LD_{50} for whole body radiation injury.
       Whole body exposure to this and smaller doses may result in intestinal
       injury amongst other effects.

a T— Anaemia, vitamin deficiencies, diarrhoea, steatorrhoea and weight loss
       may result from intestinal malabsorption.
b T— Any disorder which produces stagnation of bowel contents, such as
       multiple diverticula, strictures or a surgical intestinal bypass may produce
       the 'blind-loop' syndrome.
c F— Broad spectrum antibiotics which control the overgrowth of gram
       negative organisms are more appropriate as a short term form of
       treatment.
d T— The Schilling test reveals a lower than normal excretion of vitamin B_{12}
       which does not improve with the addition of intrinsic factor.

a F— It occurs in the terminal ileum between 50 and 100 cm from the
       ileocaecal valve.
b T— This is a developmental anomaly in which the vitello-intestinal duct fails
c T   to close at its intestinal end. All coats of intestinal wall are present and
       there may also be a fibrous cord or, rarely, a fistulous tract between the
       umbilicus and the diverticulum.
d F— Bleeding due to peptic ulceration arising from heterotopic gastric tissue
       is the commonest complication. The next commonest is intestinal
       obstruction usually caused by volvulus of the gut around the fibrous
       band attached to the umbilicus. Diverticulitis occurs in less than 25 per
       cent of symptomatic cases. Excision of the diverticulum is only
       recommended in symptomatic cases.

XII Colon, Rectum and Anus

240   **Diverticular disease of the colon:**
a   Is most common in the tropics.   ( )
b   Increases in incidence with advancing age.   ( )

c   Is associated with hypertrophied muscle in the sigmoid   ( )
colon.

d   Is precancerous.   ( )

241   **Diverticular disease of the colon:**
a   Is usually asymptomatic.   ( )

b   Often presents with lower abdominal pain.   ( )

c   May present with severe rectal haemorrhage.   ( )

d   May present with peritonitis.   ( )

242   **Uncomplicated diverticular disease of the colon:**
a   Can be most effectively treated with a low residue diet.   ( )
b   Can be most effectively treated with a high residue diet.   ( )

c   Frequently requires surgical resection of the sigmoid colon.   ( )

d   May require long term antibiotic therapy.   ( )

a   F— There is a very low incidence in tropical countries.
b   T— It is rare below 35 years and the majority of Western people have colonic
         diverticula by the age of 65.
c   T— In diverticular disease higher pressures than usual are developed in the
         sigmoid colon and this is associated with hypertrophy of the circular
         muscle coat. Diverticula of mucous membrane develop at sites where
         blood vessels pierce the muscle wall.
d   F— Both colonic cancer and diverticular disease are common in Western
         countries, they therefore frequently coexist. However, no causative
         relationship has been shown to exist between them.

a   T— Uncomplicated and asymptomatic diverticular disease is present in more
         than half of the population over 50 years of age.
b   T— Occlusion of the neck of a diverticulum leads to inflammation and
         oedema in the wall of the bowel which then occludes neighbouring
c   T   diverticula. The sigmoid colon becomes tender and pericolic inflamma-
         tion may occur with the formation of abscesses. These may resolve but
d   T   perforation into the peritoneal cavity, or an adjacent viscus, producing
         peritonitis or an internal fistula may occur. Occult rectal bleeding is
         frequently present during these attacks of inflammation and occasionally
         severe haemorrhage is seen.

a   F— Recent evidence suggests that a high bulk diet, containing large amounts
b   T   of unabsorbed fibre, will increase the faecal bulk, reduce the colonic
         pressures and halt the progression of the pathological process. A low
         bulk diet may increase colonic pressures and cause the disease to progress.
c   F— Surgery should be reserved for the complications of diverticular disease
         and those cases in which the diagnosis of colonic cancer cannot be excluded.
d   F— There is no evidence that prophylactic antibiotics will reduce the attacks
         of inflammation.

243   In ulcerative colitis:

a   The colonic mucosa demonstrates multiple wide ulcers and   (   )
      inflammatory changes.

b   There may be fibrosis of the colonic wall.   (   )

c   Colonic pseudopolyps are a feature of the early stages of   (   )
      the disease.

d   Extensive inflammatory changes also occur in the ileum.   (   )

244   In patients with ulcerative colitis a barium enema examination:

a   Should not be performed unless the disease is quiescent.   (   )

b   Often demonstrates a smooth and thinned colon.   (   )
c   Is of value in confirming the presence of proctitis.   (   )
d   Is necessary for the patients' future medical or surgical   (   )
      management.

245   Surgical treatment of ulcerative colitis:

a   Is usually by subtotal colectomy.   (   )

b   Is usually undertaken as an emergency measure.   (   )

c   May reduce the risk of colonic cancer.   (   )

d   Is often indicated for colitis confined to the recto-sigmoid   (   )
      region.

a　T— This is the fundamental pathological change, the aetiology of which is unknown.
b　T— Repeated attacks of inflammation thin the mucosal surface and extend the inflammatory process into the muscularis mucosae and eventually the muscular layers of the colonic walls. Fibrosis, resulting in shortening and stricture formation, may then occur.
c　F— Pseudopolyps are the result of repeated attacks of inflammation and ulceration and may be regarded as abnormal regeneration of colonic mucosa.
d　F— Much attention was given to an associated mild ileitis and it was thought that this represented an extension of the colonic disease to the small bowel. It is now thought more likely that it results from backwash of abnormal colonic contents through an incompetent ileocaecal valve.

a　F— Though it is dangerous to perform this examination in patients suffering from acute and severe forms of the disease it can be performed safely at other times.
b　T— Lack of haustration and a decreased colonic calibre indicate chronic
c·　F　colitis. It is usually difficult to estimate the extent of mucosal ulceration
d　T　and inflammation particularly of the rectum. The demonstration of chronic colitis with stenotic areas or suspected carcinoma is helpful when considering future management.

a　F— Total proctocolectomy and permanent ileostomy is the most usual choice of operation. The rectum is affected by the disease in most patients and if it is not excised symptoms may persist or worsen.
b　F— Elective surgery is the general rule. Toxic dilatation of the colon, acute perforation and severe haemorrhage necessitate emergency surgery but fortunately these complications are rare.
c　T— In total colitis there is a cumulative risk of colonic cancer developing—initially the risk is low but after 20 years of the disease it rises at 5 per cent per annum. After 25 years there is a 40 per cent risk of developing cancer, thus prophylactic colectomy is being more frequently undertaken in longstanding cases.
d　F— Less than 5 per cent of these cases require colonic operations. There is no increased risk of malignant change developing in this form of the disease.

246 **Longterm medical management of ulcerative colitis:**
  a   Is usually indicated in patients with total colonic involvement ( )
  b   Is usually indicated in children. ( )
  c   Is effective in the majority of patients. ( )
  d   Includes intravenous pitressin in acute exacerbations. ( )

247 **Ulcerative colitis:**
  a   Is more common in males than females. ( )
  b   Appears most commonly between the ages of 20 and 30. ( )

  c   Usually presents with abdominal discomfort and diarrhoea. ( )

  d   Can usually be diagnosed on sigmoidoscopic examination. ( )

248 **Crohn's disease of the rectum:**
  a   Is associated with an anal fissure or fistula in the majority ( )
      of cases.
  b   May produce a diffuse granular proctitis. ( )

  c   Is usually associated with ileal or colonic Crohn's disease. ( )
  d   Is characterised by long periods of remission. ( )

249 **Ischaemic colitis:**
  a   Often presents with diarrhoea. ( )
  b   Often presents with rectal bleeding. ( )

  c   Is commonly situated around the splenic flexure. ( )

  d   Is often effectively managed by non-surgical means. ( )

a   F— Children, the aged, patients with total colonic involvement and those
b   F   patients with severe attacks are all in a 'high risk' category wherein
c   T   relapses are frequent. Medical management is generally unsatisfactory in
d   F   these groups of patients. The remainder can be managed medically with
         symptomatic measures such as sedatives, anti-diarrhoeal drugs, vitamins
         and iron. Steroid enemata are of use in the acute attack and these may be
         supplemented by systemic steroids or ACTH for a short time.

a   F— There is an increased incidence in females (1.5 : 1).
b   T— Though the majority of patients present in early adult life, increasing
         numbers of patients are now presenting in old age.
c   T— These two symptoms together with rectal bleeding are by far the most
         common. Fever, joint effusions and pain, uveitis and erythema nodosum
         are associated symptoms in a minority of cases.
d   T— Almost all cases of ulcerative colitis have an associated proctitis, and
         sigmoidoscopy shows a granular oedematous mucosa which is friable and
         bleeds easily. Rectal biopsies will confirm the diagnosis.

a   T— Three-quarters of these patients have one of these lesions.

b   T— But the granulomatous infiltration of the submucosa more frequently
         causes patchy mucosal nodularity and ulceration.
c   T— Isolated rectal involvement is rarely encountered.
d   F— The disease is progressive, in contrast to nonspecific proctitis.

a   F— Diarrhoea is not an early feature. The ischaemic mucosa becomes
b   T   oedematous and ulcerates. This produces significant blood loss into the
         bowel lumen and lower abdominal pain. The pathogenesis is frequently
         obscure for often no occlusion can be found in the appropriate colonic
         vessels.
c   T— Though all parts of the colon may be affected the splenic flexure is the
         area most commonly involved.
d   T— Many patients may be managed by close observation, blood and fluid
         replacement and antibiotic therapy. A barium enema will demonstrate
         localised oedema of the bowel wall in the early stages. Late ischaemic
         strictures may develop and require surgical relief.

250 **A volvulus of the colon:**
a Most frequently occurs in Eastern Europe and Africa. ( )

b Most frequently occurs on the right side and includes the ( )
caecum.

c Usually produces abdominal distension which is most ( )
marked on the left side.

d May be effectively treated without resorting to laparotomy. ( )

251 **Hirschsprung's disease:**
a Is the result of acquired aganglionosis of the large bowel. ( )

b Usually becomes evident in early adult life. ( )

c Can usually be diagnosed on a barium enema. ( )

d Can usually be managed by dietary means. ( )

252 **Colonic polyps:**
a Are associated with colonic cancer. ( )

b May be hereditary. ( )

c Should not be removed if they are asymptomatic. ( )

d Are usually hyperplastic. ( )

a   **T—**   There is a high incidence in the Western World amongst institutionalised patients, but the highest rates are reported from Eastern Europe and Africa where high bulk diets have been blamed for producing colonic distension.

b   **F—**   Only 15 per cent of cases involve the caecum. Most of the remainder occur in the sigmoid colon where a redundant loop usually rotates on the sigmoid mesocolon.

c   **T—**   The patient presents with colicky lower abdominal pain, vomiting and gross asymmetrical distension of the abdomen. In sigmoid volvulus this is maximal on the left side.

d   **T—**   Unless there are signs of colonic strangulation the patient should be placed in the knee—elbow position (this may itself untwist the loop) and sigmoidoscoped, after which a flatus tube is gently introduced into the twisted loop to decompress. Failure to achieve this satisfying result indicates that surgical reduction or resection is required.

a   **F—**   This is a congenital condition in which aganglionosis of the rectum and part of the colon results in lack of peristaltic activity and some degree of large bowel obstruction.

b   **F—**   Most patients with this complaint have some degree of constipation in the neonatal period. Only a few cases will present in later life.

c   **T—**   The barium enema reveals dilatation of the normal colon proximal to the aganglionic segment which is of normal diameter. Diagnosis can be confirmed by a rectal biopsy which reveals the absence of a myenteric nerve plexus.

d   **F—**   Resection or bypass of the aganglionic segment must be performed. This is frequently preceded by a colostomy.

a   **T—**   In 10 per cent of resected colonic cancers there are neighbouring benign polyps. There is controversy about the exact relationships of benign polyps to neoplasia.

b   **T—**   Familial polyposis is inherited as a Mendelian dominant. It is a premalignant condition and neoplasia can only be avoided by total colectomy before the age of 20.

c   **F—**   Polyps occur in 10 to 20 per cent of the adult population and many are symptomless. However, neoplasia will arise in a proportion of polyps, therefore those that are sessile, greater than 2 cm, bleeding or apparently infiltrating should be removed as a prophylactic measure.

d   **F—**   Adenomatous polyps are the commonest tumours but juvenile polyps and hyperplastic polyps are not infrequently encountered.

253 **Villous papillomata of the large bowel:**

a Can usually be diagnosed by inspection and palpation. ( )

b Are more common on the right side of the colon. ( )

c May cause renal failure. ( )

d Rarely become malignant. ( )

254 **A right sided colonic cancer frequently presents with:**

a Anaemia. ( )

b Intestinal obstruction. ( )

c Rectal bleeding. ( )

d An abdominal mass. ( )

255 **A left sided colonic cancer frequently presents with:**

a Anaemia. ( )

b Intestinal obstruction. ( )

c Rectal bleeding. ( )

d Abdominal pain. ( )

256 **Curative cancer surgery of the colon necessitates:**

a Total excision of all neoplastic tissue. ( )

b Excision of all neighbouring related lymph nodes in
continuity. ( )

c Early control of the arterial supply to the tumour to
prevent blood-borne metastases during manipulation. ( )

d A routine 'second look' laparotomy to detect and treat
early recurrence. ( )

a T— These are velvety soft polypoid tumours which frequently spread to
b F surround the bowel lumen. Areas of malignant change can be recognised
by surface ulceration or areas of induration. 90 per cent of the tumours
occur in the rectum and distal half of the sigmoid colon.

c T— Occasionally the loss of mucus from these tumours is so excessive
(amounting to 3 litres or more per day) that hypokalaemia, hyponatraemia,
dehydration and renal failure occur.

d F— Whilst the majority of these tumours are benign, they have a very high
malignant potential. Invasive carcinoma has been reported in up to 40
per cent of these lesions.

a T— The general pattern of symptomatology of right sided colonic cancers is
b F determined by (i) their relatively long distance from the anus, and
c F (ii) the fluid bowel contents of the right side of the colon. Bleeding does
d T occur from these cancers but it is well mixed with the stool, frequently
passing unnoticed by the patient until anaemia is present. Because the
bowel contents of the right colon are fluid, intestinal obstruction is rare
and the tumour frequently enlarges to become palpable or indeed visible
on abdominal examination.

a F— The left side of the colon is narrower than the right, nearer to the anus
b T and its contents are more solid, thus rectal bleeding is usually overt and
c T noticed by the patient. The tumour frequently causes a degree of
d T obstruction which produces lower abdominal pain and pencil like stools
or frank obstruction. Thus the presentation of patients with left sided
cancers is frequently earlier than patients with right sided cancers.
Anaemia is a less common presentation in left sided lesions.

a T— In order to remove the likeliest foci of spread of malignant cells.
b T

c F— In order to diminish the risk of tumour cell embolisation the veins
draining the region of the growth are ligated before mobilisation of the
malignancy begins.

d F— This procedure, though it possesses theoretical advantages, is not yet
widely used. It remains to be demonstrated whether any improvement
in survival is sufficient to outweigh the morbidity and mortality of the
second procedure.

257   **Surgical excision of a colonic cancer:**
a   Is the only mode of cure.   (   )

b   May be inferior in terms of cure rate to radiotherapy.   (   )

c   Should not be attempted in the presence of widespread   (   )
     metastases.
d   Is complicated by anastomotic recurrences.   (   )

258   **The survival of treated patients with large bowel cancer
       depends on:**
a   The absence of lymph node metastasis.   (   )
b   The degree of differentiation of the cancer.   (   )
c   Whether the primary is right or left sided.   (   )
d   The involvement of other organs.   (   )

259   **The early diagnosis of rectal cancer may be most reliably
       achieved by:**
a   Rectal and sigmoidoscopic examination.   (   )

b   Barium enema examination.   (   )

c   Faecal occult blood estimations.   (   )
d   Detailed investigation of all patients with iron deficiency   (   )
     anaemia.

a T— It succeeds in curing 70 per cent of cases where the tumour is confined to the bowel wall and 30 per cent of those where lymph node metastases are noted.

b F— Radiotherapy is used in some centres as an adjunct to surgery for rectal cancer but the adenocarcinoma is relatively insensitive to radiation. It is not possible to safely give curative doses of radiation to the intestinal tract.

c F— Removal of an obstructing, bleeding, painful lesion is in most cases the most effective palliation for incurable cancer of the colon.

d T— Intraluminal scatter of neoplastic cells is increased during surgical manipulation of the bowel. This produces a number of recurrences at the anastomotic site.

a T— The status of the lymph nodes is a most important determinant of
b T   survival, for when cancer is present in the nodes, the survival rate drops
c T   to half that of a comparable tumour without nodes. Anaplastic tumours
d T   have the worst prognosis and the prognosis worsens if the tumour has spread through the bowel wall, particularly if it spreads extraserosally to involve other organs. There appears to be an improved survival in comparable right sided tumours — possibly due to the relative ease with which radical resection can be performed.

a T— 50 per cent of all large bowel tumours lie within reach of the sigmoidoscope.

b F— The capacious rectum does not readily yield its secrets to the radiologists — a sigmoidoscopy is essential before this investigation. The examination is time-consuming and, when regularly repeated, exposes the patient to an undue radiation hazard.

c F— Benign causes of faecal blood loss are very common.

d T— This will include full investigation of the gastrointestinal tract including sigmoidoscopy and possibly a barium enema examination.

260   Rectal cancer:

a   Is usually of squamous cell origin.   (   )

b   Usually metastasises by lymphatic spread.   (   )

c   Frequently presents with faecal impaction.   (   )

d   Frequently requires a barium enema for accurate diagnosis.   (   )

261   Rectal bleeding:

a   Which is bright red and occurring on defaecation is usually   (
     arising from the anal canal.

b   Which is dark and mixed with the stool is arising from the   (
     rectum or above.

c   Should be investigated by a sigmoidoscopic examination in   (
     all cases.

d   Should be investigated by a barium enema examination in   (
     all cases.

262   Internal haemorrhoids:

a   Usually cause pruritis.   (

b   Are often associated with intense pain.   (

c   Often become infected.   (
d   Will often resolve after conservative treatment.   (

263   An anal fistula:

a   Is usually a congenital condition.   (
b   Often presents with pruritis.   (

c   May be associated with chronic colonic inflammation.   (

d   Can be successfully treated with a low residue diet.   (

a F— The vast majority are adenocarcinomata.
b T— Lymphatic spread to pararectal and inferior mesenteric nodes is common. Venous spread also occurs and results in liver metastases.
c F— Obstruction is a very rare symptom in this condition. It usually presents with rectal bleeding, the passage of slime rectally or a sensation of constant rectal fullness.
d F— Many of the neoplasms can be palpated by digital examination. Barium enema examinations will demonstrate associated colonic pathology but are imprecise in the examination of the rectum.

a T— In these cases the blood is not mixed with the stool.

b T— Decomposition of the blood and some mixing with the stool occurs when bleeding is from the rectum or above.
c T— If the history suggests anal canal bleeding and proctosigmoidoscopy confirms this and verifies that there is no other cause in the lowest 25 cm
d F   of the gastrointestinal tract then barium enema need not be undertaken. However, a barium enema is necessary if the sigmoidoscopy is normal.

a T— They cause prolapse and thus produce irritation of the anal mucosa. Some mucous discharge follows and the perianal skin becomes excoriated and pruritic.
b F— Uncomplicated internal haemorrhoids are usually painless. Internal haemorrhoidal thrombosis produces severe anal pain which may not be relieved until haemorrhoidectomy is performed. External haemorrhoidal thrombosis is common and very painful for 3 to 5 days.
c F— This is an unusual complication.
d T— Attention to bowel habit by the prescription of a high bulk diet will help minor haemorrhoids to regress.

a F— This is an acquired condition usually arising from infected anal glands.
b T— The discharging sinus results in maceration of the perianal skin and pruritis.
c T— 30 per cent of patients with colonic Crohn's disease also possess anal fissures or fistulae. There is a high incidence also in chronic ulcerative colitis.
d F— Only surgical excision of all the sinus tract will result in cure.

264 **An anal fissure:**
  a   Is an ulcer of the anal mucosa.   (   )
  b   Usually lies anteriorly.   (   )
  c   Is more common in men.   (   )
  d   Can usually be treated conservatively.   (   )

265 **Perianal abscesses:**
  a   Commence in the anal wall.   (   )
  b   Have the same aetiology as ischiorectal abscesses.   (   )
  c   Are effectively treated by antibiotics.   (   )

  d   May result in a fistula-in-ano.   (   )

266 **Rectal prolapse:**
  a   Is commonly seen in infants.   (   )
  b   Is commonly seen in the elderly.   (   )

  c   Is often associated with poor anal tone.   (   )

  d   May in some cases be successfully treated by haemorrhoid-   (   )
      ectomy.

267 **Carcinoma of the anus:**
  a   Is generally an adenocarcinoma.   (   )
  b   Readily spreads to the inguinal lymph nodes.   (   )
  c   Has a similar prognosis to rectal carcinoma.   (   )
  d   Should usually be treated by an abdominoperineal   (   )
      resection of rectum.

a   T—   It is a linear ulcer of the anal canal usually lying posteriorly. It causes
b   F   intense pain during defaecation and is more common in women.
c   F
d   T—   The majority will heal with a laxative and local anaesthetic cream but if
              this fails a firm digital stretch under anaesthesia is usually curative. It is
              important to remember that the condition is common in Crohn's disease
              and that it may be confused with a squamous cell cancer of the anal
              canal.

a   T—   Both ischiorectal and perianal abscesses usually arise from inter-
b   T   sphincteric abscesses arising from infected anal glands.
c   F—   Antibiotics will not resolve established abscesses; early incision and
              drainage is required.
d   T—   If the infection does not completely resolve, it is likely that a fistula-in-
              ano will result.

a   T—   The disease commonly occurs in both age groups. It is particularly
b   T   common amongst elderly childless women. In infants it is fortunately not
              a chronic condition.
c   T—   This is most usual in the elderly and is associated with faecal
              incontinence.
d   T—   For mild degrees of prolapse in the elderly a mucosal resection is
              sufficient treatment; other patients may need the insertion of a
              Thiersch wire around the anus; occasionally some form of rectal
              fixation is required.

a   F—   Squamous cell carcinoma is far more common.
b   T—   It reaches these nodes via the lymphatics of the perianal skin.
c   T—   There is an overall 5 year survival rate of 40 per cent in both neoplasms.
d   T—   This allows wide excision of the perianal lymphatics. The inguinal nodes
              should be carefully observed and excised if metastases are suspected.

XIII The Liver

268 Bile:
a Is secreted by the liver only after the ingestion of food. ( )
b Is secreted at the rate of 200 to 400 ml per day. ( )
c Secretion is reduced after cholecystectomy. ( )

d Contains cholecystokinin. ( )

269 Bilirubin:
a Is synthesised from cholesterol. ( )

b Is conjugated in the liver. ( )

c Is excreted into the bowel where it forms urobilinogen. ( )

d May be formed from reabsorbed urobilinogen. ( )

270 A patient with chronic liver failure characteristically presents with:
a Tremors. ( )
b Disorders of consciousness. ( )

c Palmar erythema. ( )
d A cold collapsed peripheral circulation. ( )

271 The diagnosis of chronic liver disease may be helped by serum estimations of:
a Alkaline phosphatase. ( )

b Creatine phosphokinase. ( )
c Glutamic pyruvic transaminase (SGPT). ( )
d Glutamic oxaloacetic transaminase (SGOT). ( )

a F— The liver continually secretes bile at the rate of 600 to 800ml/day.
b F   Food intake has very little effect on biliary secretion.
c F— The gallbladder performs a storage function and is non-secretory. Its removal does not affect the biliary secretion of the liver.
d F— This intestinal hormone is released by the duodenal mucosa after the entry of food into the duodenum. It causes the gallbladder to contract and the sphincter of Oddi to relax.

a F— It is formed from the breakdown of haemoglobin by cells of the reticulo-endothelial system.
b T— It is transported, bound to albumin, to the liver and there combined with glucuronic acid to form conjugated bilirubin.
c T— Conjugated bilirubin is broken down by intestinal bacteria to form urobilinogen.
d T— Half of the urobilinogen is reabsorbed from the intestinal tract and reconverted to bilirubin in the liver.

a T— There is a coarse tremor of voluntary muscle, in advanced liver failure.
b T— This ranges from confusion to coma. It is exacerbated by a high protein intake or a gastrointestinal bleed because of the rise in the circulating undetoxicated protein products.
c T— Vasomotor tone is decreased, all peripheral pulses are easily felt and the
d F   extremities are warmer and more erythematous than normal.

a T— This enzyme is produced by bone and excreted in the bile. Therefore both bone and hepatobiliary diseases may produce a rise in its normal value.
b F— This enzyme is increased in the serum after muscle damage.
c T— Both these enzymes are widely distributed but particularly highly
d T   concentrated in the liver. Acute liver damage thus produces a rise in their serum levels.

272 **Liver failure:**

a Is the most common cause of death in patients who present ( )
with bleeding oesophageal varices.

b May be precipitated by diuretics in cirrhotic patients. ( )

c May present with personality changes. ( )

d Can be effectively treated on a temporary basis by ( )
haemodialysis.

273 **The ascites of chronic liver failure may be due to:**

a Hypoalbuminaemia. ( )
b Increased aldosterone secretion. ( )
c Hepatic vein obstruction. ( )
d Portal vein occlusion. ( )

274 **The anaemia associated with chronic liver disease may be
due to:**

a Gastrointestinal bleeding. ( )
b Decreased red cell survival. ( )
c Hypersplenism. ( )

d Deficiency of intrinsic factor. ( )

275 **Bleeding oesophageal varices:**

a Can be reliably diagnosed from a barium swallow examina- ( )
tion.

b May be treated by an oesophageal transection. ( )
c May be treated by a portocaval shunt. ( )

d May be treated by a splenectomy. ( )

a   T— The commonest cause of death is liver failure whether the varices are
        medically or surgically treated.
b   T— Disorders of fluid and electrolyte balance, particularly the hypokalaemia
        induced by most diuretics, may precipitate hepatic coma.
c   T— In the early stages alteration in mood is noted but this progresses to
        disorientation, stupor and finally coma. Associated with these signs are a
        coarse tremor, warm extremities and a mousy odour on the breath.
d   F— All treatment is supportive and aimed at reducing the nitrogenous
        content of the bowel while maintaining fluid and electrolyte balance.
        There is no evidence that haemodialysis, exchange transfusion or liver
        perfusion achieves better results.

a   T— All these factors play a part but the most important is hepatic venous
b   T   obstruction and the raised intrahepatic pressures that follow. Ascites
c   T   rarely follows an isolated portal vein occlusion.
d   T

a   T— Gastrointestinal bleeding from either oesophageal varices or duodenal
b   T   ulceration is common in cirrhotics. There is also a decreased red cell
c   T   survival time. Hypersplenism often accompanies the splenic enlargement
        of portal hypertension and results in a depression of all blood elements.
d   F— This is not present.

a   F— The history of painless vomiting of large quantities of fresh blood leads
        to an accurate diagnosis in most cases. Barium swallow and meal should
        be performed and will reveal positive evidence of varices in over 90 per
        cent of affected patients. Oesophagogastroscopy is essential to
        demonstrate whether the varices are the cause of the haemorrhage.
b   T— Transection will stop variceal bleeding for a period of time but bleeding
c   T   tends to recur earlier than when a portocaval shunt is undertaken. The
        surgical mortality is similar in both procedures, being about 40 per cent.
d   F— This produces a very temporary reduction in portal pressure and
        bleeding soon recurs.

276   Portal hypertension:

a   Is due to extrahepatic causes in approximately 50 per cent   (   )
of cases.

b   Most commonly presents in the third decade.   (   )

c   Which is associated with cirrhosis is due to post-sinusoidal   (   )
obstruction.

d   Does not usually affect life expectancy.   (   )

**277   Emergency management of bleeding oesophageal varices
should include:**

a   Frequent enemas.   (   )

b   Infusions of hypertonic saline.   (   )

c   Large quantities of intravenous potassium.   (   )

d   Intravenous posterior pituitary extract.   (   )

278   The Sengstaken triple lumen double balloon tube:

a   Should be routinely used in the management of bleeding   (   )
oesophageal varices.

b   Has significantly reduced the mortality rate of oesophageal   (   )
haemorrhage.

c   Has relatively few complications in use.   (   )

d   Is a more effective haemostatic appliance when the balloons   (   )
are inflated with very cold liquids.

279   Splenoportography:

a   Should be performed under a general anaesthetic.   (   )

b   Allows portal pressure to be estimated.   (   )

c   May demonstrate the site of portal vein obstruction.   (   )

d   Is helpful in the diagnosis of hepatic tumours.   (   )

a   F— Intrahepatic causes due to cirrhosis account for 90 per cent of cases. The major extrahepatic cause is portal vein thrombosis.
b   F— Cirrhosis takes many years to develop and thus the majority of patients are in late middle life.
c   T— The cirrhotic process particularly constricts the smallest tributaries of the hepatic veins.
d   F— The 5 year survival is very poor; only 5 to 10 per cent of patients with cirrhosis and portal hypertension survive this period.

a   T— Together with oral neomycin and nasogastric aspiration these will reduce the risk of hepatic coma arising from bacterial action on the nitrogenous bowel contents.
b   F— Fresh blood will almost certainly be required. Cirrhotic patients have a marked increase in total body sodium and thus saline infusions should only be given after exceptional losses.
c   T— Hypokalaemic alkalosis frequently accompanies bleeding oesophageal varices.
d   T— This produces a temporary drop in portal pressure, sufficient in some cases to stop the bleeding.

a   T— This tube has a limited role in providing a very temporary means of stopping massive haemorrhage prior to surgery. Rebleeding frequently
b   F   follows withdrawal of the balloon. Oesophageal perforation, aspiration pneumonia and asphyxia have been reported after its use.
c   F
d   F— It is not possible to circulate fluid through these balloons and it is unlikely that local hypothermia stops gastro-oesophageal bleeding.

a   F— The technique is usually performed under local anaesthesia via a needle introduced percutaneously into the splenic pulp.
b   T— There is a close correlation between the splenic pulp pressure and that in the portal vein. In health this varies between 8 and 12 cm of water.
c   T— It may differentiate between intra- and extra-hepatic causes of portal hypertension.
d   T— Space occupying lesions of the liver are well demonstrated by the abnormal intrahepatic venous pattern.

280   A portocaval shunt:

a   Should, where possible, be performed in patients with   (   )
oesophageal varices before bleeding occurs (prophylacti-
cally).

b   Carries the risk of precipitating liver failure.   (   )
c   Prevents further haemorrhage from varices in the large   (   )
majority of patients.
d   Is most applicable to cases with extrahepatic portal   (   )
occlusion.

281   A liver abscess:

a   Is commonly associated with gallstones.   (   )
b   Typically produces a firm enlarged tender liver.   (   )
c   Is usually accompanied by jaundice.   (   )
d   Commonly produces a right sided pleural effusion.   (   )

282   Hydatid cysts of the liver:

a   Are frequently asymptomatic.   (   )
b   Are commoner in rural areas.   (   )

c   Require surgical removal.   (   )
d   May produce jaundice and fever.   (   )

283   Liver cancer:

a   Is commoner in patients with cirrhosis.   (   )

b   Often presents with ascites.   (   )

c   Has an increased incidence in sheep farmers.   (   )
d   Produces measurable serum levels of a fetal protein.   (   )

a   F— There is no evidence to suggest that this form of 'prophylactic' shunt surgery improves longevity. However, once the varices have bled then successful shunt surgery is followed by a 5 year survival of approximately 50 per cent of patients. 'Medical' management of this group results in almost 100 per cent mortality over the same period.

b   T— Liver failure is the commonest major complication after shunt surgery,

c   T   and may result in death. Rebleeding however does not commonly occur.

d   F— This rare cause of portal hypertension can only be treated by a spleno-renal or mesocaval portosystemic anastomosis.

a   T— The commonest cause in Britain of a liver abscess is cholangitis

b   T   associated with gallstones in the common bile duct. The patient is

c   T   pyrexial with pain in the right upper quadrant due to an enlarged tender

d   T   liver. Jaundice is almost always present and an ipsilateral pleural effusion is common. X-rays show elevation of the diaphragm, blood cultures are frequently positive and ultrasonography or liver scanning may demonstrate the lesion. Antibiotics and surgical drainage are required.

a   T— In its life cycle, the echinococcus has dog as its primary host and sheep,

b   T   cattle or man as its intermediate host. Thus the disease is commoner in rural areas. Infestation occurs by the ingested embryos passing through the portal vein to the liver where they reproduce to form multilocular cysts — many of which are asymptomatic.

c   T— Once the diagnosis is confirmed (by X-rays, liver scans, Casoni and other

d   T   serological tests) the cyst should be removed for rupture of the cyst may occur and cause fever, jaundice and possibly anaphylactic shock due to the dissemination of multiple daughter cysts.

a   T— About 5 per cent of all cirrhotics will develop liver cancer, and cirrhotics account for 75 per cent of all liver cancers.

b   T— The presentation is sudden, with rapidly progressive ascites, weight loss, jaundice and pain in the right hypochondrium.

c   F— Hydatid disease, but not liver cancer, is commoner in sheep farmers.

d   T— All the liver function tests may be abnormal, particularly the alkaline phosphatase. Alpha fetoprotein is noted in more than 50 per cent of the patients with primary liver cancer.

XIV Extrahepatic Biliary System, Spleen and Pancreas

284   Acute cholecystitis:

a   Is almost invariably related to the presence of gallstones.   (   )

b   Usually presents with biliary colic.   (   )

c*   Is often associated with jaundice.   (   )

d   Is characterised by a pyrexia in the early hours of the disease.   (   )

285   Acute cholecystitis should usually be treated by:

a   Nasogastric suction and intravenous fluids.   (   )
b   Antibiotic therapy.   (   )
c   Urgent cholecystectomy.   (   )
d   Cholecystostomy.   (   )

286   Biliary obstruction:

a   May be diagnosed by decreased bromsulphthalein (BSP) clearance.   (   )

b   May be diagnosed by decreased biliary excretion of rose bengal dye.   (   )

c   May be diagnosed by an oral cholecystogram.   (   )

d   May cause a prolonged prothrombin time.   (   )

a T— More than 95 per cent of the patients with acute cholecystitis have gallstones. Acute cholecystitis usually follows blockage of the cystic duct with a stone.
b T— The pain is felt in the right upper quadrant and often radiates to the back, becoming continuous in 2 or 3 hours. Reflex vomiting is usually present.
c T— A slightly raised bilirubin (about 2 to 3 mg/100ml (30 to 45 μmol/l)) is frequently found in acute cholecystitis. Bilirubin values above this level usually indicate a stone in the common bile duct.
d F— Cystic duct calculus obstruction often relieves itself before the distended gallbladder becomes secondarily infected. Where this does not occur cholecystitis develops and pyrexia develops after 24 to 36 hours.

a T— The majority of cases will respond to conservative treatment. This is
b T   followed by an elective cholecystectomy, 2 or 3 months later. Although
c F   an increasing number of surgeons believe urgent cholecystectomy to be
d F   desirable, it is a more demanding surgical exercise and not to be generally recommended. Cholecystostomy is only occasionally indicated when acute cholecystitis does not resolve after conservative management and cholecystectomy is judged too hazardous.

a F— BSP is cleared from the blood by the liver and the test is used to appraise hepatocellular function. The presence of biliary obstruction invalidates the investigation.
b T— This synthetic dye is cleared from the blood stream by the liver and excreted in the bile. When labelled with I^{131} its excretion can be estimated by radiation counters.
c F— The contrast media are not concentrated in the bile when the serum bilirubin is above 3 mg/100 ml (51μmol/l) and so no radiological diagnosis is possible by this technique.
d T— The lack of bile salts in the intestinal tract interferes with the absorption of vitamin K_1 which is essential for prothrombin synthesis. This defect may be overcome by an intramuscular injection of vitamin K_1.

287 Gallstones:

a   Have an incidence which increases with age. ( )

b   Are more frequent in females. ( )

c   Usually contain a predominance of calcium carbonate. ( )

d   Are formed in bile which is supersaturated with bile acids. ( )

288 The presence of stones in the common bile duct:

a   Is commonly associated with a long history of dyspepsia. ( )

b   Is invariably associated with jaundice. ( )

c   Must be considered during every cholecystectomy. ( )

d   Occasionally requires treatment by choledochoduodenostomy. ( )

289 Stones in the common bile duct:

a   Are present in nearly 50 per cent of cases of cholecystitis. ( )

b   Often give rise to jaundice, fever and biliary colic. ( )

c   Are usually accompanied by progressive jaundice. ( )

d   Are not usually associated with a distended gallbladder. ( )

290 Oral cholecystography:

a   May not opacify the gallbladder when gallstones are present. ( )

b   Is frequently unsatisfactory if intestinal absorption is diminished ( )

c   Will only opacify the gallbladder when the serum bilirubin is less than 3 mg/100 ml (51μmol/l). ( )

d   Demonstrates evidence of cholelithiasis in less than 70 per cent of affected patients. ( )

a T— 15 to 20 per cent of adults over the age of 40 have gallstones. Females
b T   are much more commonly affected than males, particularly in middle
      life.
c F— The majority of stones have cholesterol as their major component. It is
      mixed with calcium carbonate and bilirubinate.
d F— Gallstones tend to form in abnormal bile which is supersaturated with
      cholesterol. The cause of this abnormality is not yet established.

a T— This association tends to distinguish the condition from other causes of
      jaundice such as hepatitis and neoplasia of the pancreas or bile ducts.
b F— Only about 75 per cent of cases of choledocholithiasis produce jaundice.
c T— Especially if the common bile duct is dilated, if the gallbladder contains
      multiple small stones or if the operative cholangiogram demonstrates
      filling defects within the common bile duct.
d T— Though the simpler procedure of choledochotomy is sufficient in the
      majority of cases, it may be indicated if there is a stenosis of the ampulla
      of Vater or if residual intrahepatic calculi exist.

a F— Approximately 10 per cent of patients with cholecystitis have stones in
      the common bile duct. These stones usually originate in the gallbladder.
b T— This is a classical presentation (Charcot's triad).
c F— The jaundice is typically intermittent and thus distinguishable from the
      jaundice of a malignant obstruction which is progressive.
d T— The gallbladder is fibrotic and non-distensible due to accompanying
      chronic cholecystitis. Courvoisier first noted that an obstructive jaundice
      associated with an enlarged palpable gallbladder is usually due to
      malignancy.

a T— Failure of opacification of the biliary tree and gallbladder is frequently
b T   due to cystic duct obstruction by a gallstone or chronic cholecystitis.
      Lack of absorption of the oral medium, or failure of the liver to
c T   concentrate it when liver function is impaired, may produce this effect.

d F— Oral cholecystography is one of the most reliable contrast radiological
      techniques of the gastrointestinal tract. It will produce evidence of
      gallbladder disease in more than 90 per cent of affected patients.

291 In severe jaundice diagnostic evidence of an extrahepatic
obstruction of the biliary tract may be gained by:
a Intravenous cholangiography. ( )

b A barium meal. ( )
c Endoscopic retrograde cholangiography. ( )
d Percutaneous transhepatic cholangiography. ( )

292 **Internal biliary fistulae:**
a Most commonly arise as a consequence of cholecystitis. ( )
b Most commonly occur between the gallbladder and the ( )
duodenum.
c Can result in intestinal obstruction. ( )

d Are in most cases fatal complications. ( )

293 **Carcinoma of the gallbladder:**
a Is usually a squamous cell neoplasm. ( )
b Is more common in men. ( )
c Is usually associated with gallstones. ( )
d Has a relatively poor prognosis. ( )

294 **Hypersplenism:**
a Results in anaemia, leucopenia and thrombocytopenia. ( )

b Only occurs in the presence of a large spleen. ( )

c Frequently follows liver cirrhosis. ( )

d May be diagnosed by bone marrow biopsy. ( )

a   F—   If the serum bilirubin is above 4 to 5 mg/100ml (68 to 85μmol/l) no visualisation of the biliary tract will be achieved.

b   T—   A barium meal is essential in the investigation of obstructive jaundice as

c   T   it will yield information about the head of the pancreas and the

d   T   ampullary region. Retrograde cannulation of the ampulla allows cholangiography to be achieved directly and is occasionally of great diagnostic value. Percutaneous transhepatic cholangiography may yield valuable information prior to laparotomy if the intrahepatic bile ducts are obstructed and distended.

a   T—   By far the commonest cause is an inflamed gallbladder becoming adherent

b   T   to a neighbouring viscus and the contained gallstones eroding into this viscus. More than 75 per cent of these fistulae are between the gallbladder

c   T   and duodenum. Occasionally the passage of gallstones into the intestinal tract results in intestinal obstruction, usually in the terminal ileum, the narrowest part of the intestinal tract.

d   F—   Though cholangitis may occasionally be a complication, it is probable that many such fistulae close after the gallstones have left the gallbladder.

a   F—   The majority are adenocarcinomas and are much more common in

b   F   females. The incidence is highest in the elderly and more than 90 per cent

c   T   of cases are associated with gallstones. It is widely believed, but not

d   T   proven, that calculous cholecystitis is an aetiological factor. The symptoms are usually similar in the two conditions. The 5 year survival is less than 5 per cent — the tumour is usually advanced at the time of presentation.

a   T—   Hypersplenism produces trapping of the formed elements of the blood within the spleen and an abnormally high rate of destruction of red and white blood cells and platelets.

b   T—   Hypersplenism is always the result of a hypertrophied spleen either by inflammatory, infiltrative or congestive processes. Splenectomy usually reverses these changes.

c   T—   Any process which produces portal hypertension may result in hypersplenism.

d   T—   Increased erythropoiesis and an excess of megakaryocytes will be noted.

295 **Acute pancreatitis:**
a Has a higher incidence in alcoholics.   ( )
b Is commonly associated with the presence of gallstones.   ( )
c Occurs most commonly in diabetics.   ( )

d Becomes more severe with each recurring episode.   ( )

296 **Acute pancreatitis is characterised by:**
a A history of gallstones.   ( )

b Diffuse epigastric pain.   ( )

c Exaggerated bowel sounds.   ( )

d An elevated urinary diastase.   ( )

297 **Chronic pancreatitis:**
a Is commonly associated with alcoholism.   ( )

b Is associated with diabetes.   ( )

c May be diagnosed by the analysis of pancreatic secretions.   ( )

d May be treated by surgical procedures which decompress the pancreatic duct.   ( )

a   T— The aetiology of this condition is unknown, but biliary reflux into the

b   T   pancreatic duct and spasm of the sphincter of Oddi are thought to be

c   F   important. In Britain about half the patients have co-existing gallstones though of these only a small proportion have stones in the common bile duct. There is an increased incidence in alcoholics and in the U.S. this is the most commonly associated condition. It does not occur very commonly in diabetics.

d   F— It is usual that the first attack is the most severe. Further attacks usually decrease in severity.

a   T— In the United Kingdom gallstones are associated in approximately 40 per cent of cases. In the U.S.A. alcoholism is by far the commonest associated factor.

b   T— The pain may be slow in onset but often becomes severe, constant and radiating to the back and the left flank.

c   F— Bowel sounds are diminished or absent in severe cases because of the associated paralytic ileus.

d   T— The serum amylase is very frequently raised but often for only 24 hours or so. The urinary diastase is similarly elevated but for 1 or 2 days longer. It is thus a more useful diagnostic tool.

a   T— The fundamental cause of this condition is as obscure as that of acute pancreatitis but biliary tract disease and alcoholism are again frequently associated.

b   T— Chronic epigastric pain radiating to the back, diabetes, steatorrhoea and weight loss combine to form the classical presentation.

c   T— Diagnosis may be difficult but the enzyme content of the pancreatic secretions secreted in response to hormonal or food stimulation is frequently diminished.

d   T— Pancreatic duct obstruction is the usual cause of the progression of the disease, thus sphincteroplasty or drainage of the duct into the jejunum may be employed with moderately good results. If gallstones are present cholecystectomy should be performed.

298   Pancreatic pseudocysts:

a   Are developmental in origin.   (   )

b   Usually arise in the lesser peritoneal sac.   (   )

c   Produce a smooth epigastric mass which moves on   (   )
respiration.

d   May be effectively treated by internal drainage.   (   )

299   The Zollinger-Ellison syndrome:

a   Is the result of hypergastrinaemia.   (   )

b   Is produced by parietal cell neoplasia.   (   )

c   Includes diarrhoea and malabsorption among its presenting   (   )
features.

d   Is most effectively treated by total gastrectomy.   (   )

300   Tumours of the Zollinger-Ellison type:

a   Arise from the beta cells of the pancreas.   (   )

b   Often produce unusual duodenal ulcers.   (   )

c   Are frequently malignant.   (   )

d   Are best treated by partial pancreatectomy.   (   )

a   F—   There is usually a history of preceding pancreatitis or trauma. They arise following rupture of a pancreatic duct and the subsequent leakage of pancreatic secretions into the retroperitoneal tissues.

b   T—   They are thus commonly related to surrounding organs, the stomach, liver and colon.

c   F—   Though a smooth mass can usually be palpated, it does not move on respiration.

d   T—   Internal drainage of the cyst into the stomach or small bowel is the preferred treatment providing the cyst is not infected and its wall is well formed. Pancreatic abscesses should be drained externally.

a   T—   In this syndrome excessive amounts of gastrin are produced by non-beta

b   F   cell islet tumours of the pancreas. 50 per cent of these tumours are malignant and metastasise to lymph nodes and the liver. The tumours are frequently multiple.

c   T—   There is a very high acid secretion, more than 15 mEq (15 mmol)/hr. It is thought that this high acid secretion inactivates lipase to produce steatorrhoea and diarrhoea.

d   T—   Because of the multiplicity of the tumours in the pancreas, surgical removal of single tumours is rarely successful in reducing the gastric hypersecretory state. Removal of the 'target' organ by total gastrectomy is thus preferred.

a   F—   The tumours arise from non-beta cells of the pancreas, and, in producing high levels of gastrin, result in very high concentrations of acid in the gastric juice.

b   T—   The commonest presentation is for the patient to demonstrate recurrent duodenal ulceration after apparently adequate therapy or for peptic ulcers to appear in the second and third parts of the duodenum or in the jejunum. The diagnosis is confirmed by finding high levels of serum gastrin.

c   T—   The majority are malignant and multiple tumours are common.

d   F—   Because of the difficulty of locating these often small and multiple tumours, partial pancreatectomy is frequently unsuccessful. Total gastrectomy, by removing the end organ of the syndrome, achieves the best results.

301 **Cancer of the pancreas:**
a Produces epigastric discomfort. ( )
b Produces abdominal pain which is usually relieved by ( )
lying down.

c Frequently cannot be precisely diagnosed prior to ( )
laparotomy.

d Is usually treated by radical surgery. ( )

XV Genito-Urinary Tract

302 **Haematuria:**
a At the beginning of micturition is usually indicative of ( )
urethral pathology.
b At the end of micturition is usually due to bladder neck ( )
pathology.
c Throughout the urinary stream is typical of renal pathology. ( )
d In elderly males is usually related to benign prostatic ( )
hypertrophy.

303 **An intravenous pyelogram:**
a Yields most diagnostic information when performed on a ( )
well hydrated patient.
b Should be preceded by a plain film of the abdomen. ( )

c Normally shows incomplete filling of the ureter in any one ( )
exposure.

d Should provide evidence of the presence, if any, of lower ( )
urinary tract obstruction.

a   T— Vague abdominal pain and weight loss are the earliest signs and these
b   F   often only appear when the cancer is at an advanced stage. Later the
pain usually radiates to the back and is worse on lying down. Jaundice
frequently complicates cancer of the head of the pancreas.

c   T— The barium meal may show effacement of the greater curvature
of the stomach or the duodenal loop — but this is a late and inconstant
sign. No precise biochemical diagnostic test exists and radioisotope
scanning is imprecise. Cytology of pancreatic fluid is yielding good results
in some centres. Mesenteric arteriography may demonstrate some
tumours but at present laparotomy is the most certain method of
diagnosis.

d   F— Radical surgery can only be undertaken in a small proportion of cases
since the majority of patients have such advanced disease that only
palliative measures are possible.

a   T— This pattern of haematuria is due to a lesion situated distal to the external
sphincter.

b   T— This pattern of haematuria is caused by pathology in the region of the
bladder neck, trigone or posterior urethra.

c   T— Infection, neoplasia and blood dyscrasias should be considered.

d   T— This is the commonest cause of haematuria in elderly males. The
bleeding arises from fragile veins over the urethral surface of the gland.

a   F— Better concentration is achieved when the patient is slightly dehydrated.

b   T— This often shows the renal size and the majority of renal and ureteric
calculi.

c   T— Peristalsis of the healthy ureter ensures that it is incompletely filled by
contrast. If complete filling of the ureter is demonstrated then some
degree of ureteric obstruction should be suspected.

d   T— Films should be taken of the bladder after micturition. In the healthy
bladder there is an insignificant residue, whereas in bladder neck
obstruction there is an increased postmicturition residue.

304   Wilms' tumours:

a   Metastasise readily to the lungs.   (   )

b   Metastasise readily to the bones.   (   )

c   Are occasionally bilateral.   (   )
d   Have the worst prognosis of all childhood abdominal   (   )
      tumours.

305   Renal artery stenosis:

a   Is a common cause of hypertension.   (   )

b   Is most commonly caused by fibro-muscular hyperplasia.   (   )
c   Can usually be diagnosed on an intravenous pyelogram.   (   )

d   Should be treated by nephrectomy.   (   )

306   In renal transplantation:

a   A donor kidney may be used from a patient with malignancy   (   )
      provided there is no abdominal involvement.

b   ABO compatibility between donor and recipient does not   (   )
      have to be considered.
c   Satisfactory renal function can be expected with a warm   (   )
      ischaemic time of up to 200 minutes.

d   The characteristic signs of acute rejection include pyrexia,   (   )
      hypertension and leucocytosis.

a **T—** This embryonal neoplasm usually presents with an abdominal mass and haematuria. Pulmonary metastases are seen in more than 25 per cent of cases on presentation.

b **F—** In contradistinction to neuroblastomata and adult renal cancers, bone metastases are rare.

c **T—** Up to 6 per cent of cases have been shown to have bilateral tumours.

d **F—** Aggressive 'triple therapy' with radical excision of the primary tumour and associated lymph nodes, postoperative radiotherapy to the primary site and areas of metastasis together with postoperative Actinomycin D or Vincristine result in high cure rates (90 per cent where no metastases are present and 40 per cent where lymph node metastases have occurred).

a **F—** This uncommon cause of hypertension usually presents as an abrupt onset of hypertension in a middle aged patient. (The practice of screening all hypertensive patients for the condition by intravenous pyelography has been unproductive.)

b **F—** The commonest cause is atheromatous narrowing of the renal artery.

c **T—** A slight decrease in renal size, delay in opacification of the renal pelvis and late hyperconcentration of contrast medium (due to excessive tubular reabsorption of water) are all suggestive of the condition.

d **F—** Careful assessment of the patient's general condition including the function of the opposite kidney and the nature of the arterial occlusion lead to surgical treatment being advised in approximately half the patients. Usually this is by arterial reconstruction although nephrectomy is occasionally necessary.

a **F—** Patients with malignancy are unsuitable donors, as are the aged, patients with renal disease or hypertension. Best results are obtained when the donor organ is from a living blood relative. The most satisfactory cadaver donors are young patients dying of head injuries.

b **F—** Donor and recipient must be ABO compatible; otherwise, hyperacute rejection may occur within a few minutes.

c **F—** Maximum renal function is obtained with warm ischaemic times of under 30 minutes, if this time exceeds 100 minutes it cannot be expected and the kidney should not be transplanted.

d **T—** Acute rejection is seen during the first three months after transplantation. Some success has been achieved in treating such episodes with high doses of steroids and immunosuppressive drugs.

307 **An adenocarcinoma of the kidney:**

a Usually occurs in the 35 to 45 age group. ( )

b Usually presents with a urinary infection. ( )

c Is often indistinguishable from a renal cyst radiologically. ( )

d Frequently invades and grows along the renal artery. ( )

308 **Tumours of the renal pelvis:**

a Usually present as a mass in the loin. ( )

b Are possibly due to a urinary carcinogen. ( )

c Resemble those of the bladder in their histology. ( )
d Are best treated by a partial or total nephrectomy. ( )

309 **Ureteric calculi:**

a Often result from urinary tract infection. ( )

b Frequently cause haematuria. ( )

c Are not usually radio-opaque. ( )

d Producing ureteric colic should be surgically removed. ( )

310 **Cancer of the penis:**

a Is more common in the circumcised. ( )

b Commonly arises from the corona of glans penis. ( )

c Is usually an adenocarcinoma. ( )
d Rarely metastasises. ( )

a F— It usually occurs between the age of 50 to 70 years and it is rare before the age of 30.
b F— Haematuria, loin pain and a mass are the usual symptoms but they may be preceded by general malaise or the symptoms of a bony metastasis.
c T— The differential diagnosis from the more common condition of renal cysts may require further investigations such as selective renal angiography or ultrasound studies.
d F— The renal vein is commonly involved by the tumour growing along it and sometimes reaching the inferior vena cava where it may embolise.

a F— Although on rare occasions the tumour may block the ureter and give rise to hydronephrosis the usual presentation is with haematuria and clot colic.
b T— Tumours of the renal pelvis resemble those of the bladder in that they may be due to a urinary carcinogen.
c T— They are carcinomas arising from transitional epithelium.
d F— Their spread is by seedlings to ureter and bladder. They are therefore treated by nephrectomy and ureterectomy, the latter being extended to include an adjacent cuff of bladder wall.

a T— Infection, stasis, prolonged immobilisation and generalised metabolic diseases such as gout, hyperparathyroidism and cystinuria may cause urinary calculi.
b T— This may not be overt but urinalysis usually reveals erythrocytes in the urine.
c F— More than 90 per cent of ureteric calculi are radio-opaque. Uric acid calculi are not.
d F— Most stones measuring less than 4 mm diameter on X-ray will pass spontaneously.

a F— It is very much commoner in the uncircumcised and is commonest amongst Social Class V.
b T— This is much the commonest site where it may also be hidden by the foreskin.
c F— It is a squamous cell carcinoma.
d F— Inguinal lymph node metastases are common. Infection of the neoplasm may also produce enlarged regional nodes and care should be taken to distinguish infective from neoplastic lymph node enlargement.

311 **Carcinoma of the prostate:**
a Is commonly of squamous cell origin. ( )
b Usually originates in the periphery of the gland. ( )
c Usually presents relatively early with lower urinary tract ( )
symptoms.

d Can be readily diagnosed on rectal examination. ( )

312 **Carcinoma of the prostate:**
a Does not usually metastasise. ( )

b Usually produces an elevated serum acid phosphatase. ( )

c Can be effectively treated by hormones. ( )

d Is most effectively treated by surgery. ( )

313 **Benign prostatic hypertrophy:**
a Is the result of hyperplasia of the fibromuscular capsule of ( )
the gland.

b Results in diminished power of urination. ( )
c Results in terminal dribbling of urine. ( )
d Often presents with haematuria. ( )

a **F—** Adenocarcinoma is by far the most common form.
b **T—** Particularly in the posterior part of the capsule.
c **F—** Unfortunately symptoms are not present in the early stages of prostatic cancer. Its peripheral origin ensures that urethral involvement occurs late in the disease.
d **T—** The advanced case demonstrates a nodular diffuse hardness often with fixation to surrounding structures. The early case will present as a solitary hard nodule which must be considered carcinoma until proved otherwise.

a **F—** Metastases are very common and are often blood borne, thus the skeleton, particularly the sacrum and lumbar spine, and the lungs are frequently involved.
b **T—** Small tumours and those with a low metabolic activity may be associated with normal values.
c **T—** Bilateral orchidectomy or daily stilboestral has been frequently shown to be associated with good 10 year survival rates, regardless of the stage of the disease. However, in some patients the risks of oestrogen therapy (congestive cardiac failure and cerebral and coronary thrombosis) may be higher than the risks of the disease.
d **F—** Less than 10 per cent of patients have cancer limited to the gland and radical surgery should only be offered to fit patients with a relatively long life expectancy.

a **F—** Senile prostatic hyperplasia follows proliferation of the central peri-urethral glandular tissue. A lobular growth pattern usually involves either the median lobe beneath the bladder trigone or the lateral lobes. The peripheral capsule of the gland is displaced and compressed by this process.
b **T—** As the hyperplasia develops the prostatic urethra narrows and elongates
c **T** and a mechanical obstruction to micturition develops. The force and size
d **T** of the stream decreases. Frequency and terminal dribbling often indicate an increased residual urine and dysuria resulting from infection is common. Haematuria occurs quite commonly and results from damage to engorged urethral veins during micturition.

314 **Benign prostatic hypertrophy:**
a   Can readily be assessed on rectal examination.   (   )

b   Can be effectively treated with hormones.   (   )
c   Is most effectively treated by surgery.   (   )

d   Is a premalignant condition.   (   )

315 **Acute prostatitis:**
a   Is most commonly due to coliform organisms.   (   )

b   Often presents as an ache in the perineum.   (   )

c   May be diagnosed by rectal examination.   (   )
d   Requires bladder catheterisation as part of the treatment.   (   )

316 **Bladder cancer:**
a   May follow exposure to beta-naphthylamine.   (   )

b   Is more common in heavy smokers.   (   )
c   Is more common in females.   (   )

d   Is frequently associated with bladder schistosomiasis.   (   )

317 **Bladder cancers:**
a   Are usually adenocarcinomas.   (   )
b   Are usually ulcerating.   (   )
c   Usually present with suprapubic pain radiating to the   (   )
perineum.

d   Are usually diagnosed on excretory pyelography.   (   )

a   F— Rectal assessment of prostate size is not reliable for the median lobe is
         impalpable. (The degree of prostatic hypertrophy is not related to the
         amount of urinary obstruction. Small glands may produce obstruction
         and large glands none.)
b   F— Hormonal therapy has not yet proved satisfactory.
c   T— Though the general condition of the patient and the extent of his
         disability must always be considered.
d   F— There is no firm evidence relating benign hyperplasia with neoplasia of
         the gland.

a   T— *Escherichia coli* is the commonest organism isolated. Acute gonococcal
         prostatitis may also occur.
b   T— This is a common symptom together with dysuria, urgency and
         frequency. Fever and rigors are often present.
c   T— The prostate is diffusely enlarged and very tender.
d   F— Instrumentation of the lower urinary tract should be avoided, unless
         urinary retention is present, for bacteraemic shock may follow. Broad
         spectrum antibiotics should be prescribed for at least 2 weeks.

a   T— Industrial and laboratory use of this chemical is now very strictly
         controlled.
b   T— Although a urinary carcinogen has not yet been isolated in these patients.
c   F— It is 3 to 4 times commoner in males and occurs mainly in the sixth and
         seventh decades.
d   T— Schistosoma haematobium is thought to predispose to bladder cancer.
         There is a high incidence of bladder cancer in regions where schistosom-
         iasis is endemic.

a   F— These are rare. The commonest neoplasm is a transitional cell carcinoma
b   F   and these usually form sessile tumours which only occasionally ulcerate.
c   F— This is a sign of advanced and incurable disease. The commonest
         presenting sign is of painless intermittent haematuria which may later
         become associated with symptoms of cystitis and strangury (pain at the
         end of micturition).
d   F— The intravenous pyelogram frequently shows no disturbance of renal
         function. Only large bladder cancers will be revealed on the cystogram.
         Cystoscopy is the most reliable method of diagnosis and should be
         performed in all patients suspected of the disease.

318   Undescended testes:

a   Are often associated with inguinal herniae.   (   )

b   Usually descend at puberty.   (   )

c   Can usually be made to descend by the examiner with warm   (   )
         hands.

d   Should be treated by orchidopexy at puberty.   (   )

319   The spermatic cord contains:

a   The inferior epigastric vein.   (   )
b   The deep circumflex iliac artery.   (   )
c   The pudendal nerve.   (   )
d   The subcostal nerve.   (   )

320   Torsion of the spermatic cord:

a   Often presents with vomiting and lower abdominal pain.   (   )
b   Often produces gangrene of the testis.   (   )

c   May initially be treated effectively by non-surgical means.   (   )

d   Always requires surgical treatment.   (   )

321   Seminomas of the testis:

a   Most commonly occur before the age of 40.   (   )

b   Are usually sensitive to radiotherapy.   (   )
c   Rarely metastasise via the blood stream.   (   )
d   Generally carry a poor prognosis.   (   )

a   T— This relatively common abnormality (which occurs in 2 to 4 per cent of male children) is usually associated with a patent processus vaginalis and an inguinal hernia.

b   F— This is rare, and usually means that the original diagnosis should have been that of a retractile testis.

c   F— Undescended testes cannot be brought below the neck of the scrotum. Those that can be encouraged into the scrotum are merely retractile and not pathological.

d   F— Surgical replacement of the testis into the scrotum by the age of 6 years ensures normal spermatogenesis and may decrease the higher incidence of neoplasia that occurs in abdominal testes.

a   F— The spermatic cord is invested with external and internal spermatic fascia

b   F   together with the cremaster muscle. It contains testicular vessels, the

c   F   vas deferens, the ilio-inguinal nerve and sympathetic nerve fibres. A patent

d   F   processus vaginalis is present in those patients with an indirect inguinal hernia.

a   T— Together with the sudden onset of severe testicular pain.

b   T— This is almost inevitable unless the torsion is corrected within 12 hours.

c   T— Manual correction, by rotating the testis in the direction which is the least painful is often successful in releasing the torsion.

d   T— Fixation of the abnormally mobile testis (and its opposite number) is always indicated even if initial relief has been obtained by non-surgical means.

a   T— Though they may occur at any age more than 80 per cent occur before the age of 40.

b   T— The majority are radiosensitive and, since blood borne metastases are

c   T   less common, surgical removal of the affected testis combined with radio-

d   F   therapy to the iliac and para-aortic nodes produce 5 year survival rates of up to 90 per cent. Teratomas of the testis are less radio-sensitive, metastasise more frequently via the blood stream and have a much worse prognosis.

322 **A teratoma of the testis:**

a May contain ectodermal or endodermal but not mesodermal ( )
cells.

b Has a 5 year survival of up to 80 per cent in the teratoma ( )
differentiated (TD) variety.

c May be diagnosed by the Aschheim-Zondek pregnancy ( )
test.

d Should only be treated by radiotherapy in incurable cases. ( )

323 **Hypospadias:**

a Is the result of failure of scrotal development. ( )

b Results in the abnormal urethra opening onto the dorsum ( )
of the penis.

c Is associated with chordee. ( )

d Is associated with maldescent of the testis. ( )

XVI Lymphatic and Vascular Systems

324 **The protein content of the lymph:**

a From the liver is over 5g/100ml (50g/l). ( )
b From the periphery is 2g/100ml (20g/l). ( )
c From the gastrointestinal tract is 3 to 5g/100ml (30 to 50g/l). ( )
d In the thoracic duct is 8g/100ml (80g/l). ( )

325 **The lymphatic vessels:**

a Of most tissues bear a direct numerical relation to the ( )
vascular capillaries.

b Of the pyloric antrum pass directly to the lymphatic duct ( )
without traversing any lymph nodes.

c Drain 50 per cent of the arterial capillary filtrate. ( )

d Are almost totally responsible for the reabsorption of ( )
protein from the interstitial fluid.

a F— These tumours arise from the totipotent cells of the rete testis and may be of any germ layer, one form being usually predominant.

b T— Survival figures vary with the histological type, TD having the best prognosis while the malignant teratoma trophoblastic, MTT (which may

c T have a positive pregnancy test) has an extremely poor prognosis. The introduction of routine prophylactic radiotherapy to the para-aortic

d F nodes has, with these tumours as well as the seminoma, markedly improved survival figures.

a F— It is the result of incomplete development of the anterior urethra.

b F— In hypospadias the urethra opens onto the ventral aspect of the glans or penile shaft.

c T— In severe cases the fibrous remnant of the undeveloped urethra gives an abnormal downward curvature to the penis.

d T— This is rare but the resulting state of the external genitalia may produce a state of intersex.

a T

b T

c T

d F— Since it is a mixture of lymph from all sources, its protein content is 3 to 5g/100ml (30 to 50g/l).

a T— Rare exceptions being the central nervous system and the spleen which contain no lymphatic capillaries.

b F— This is only true of the lymph vessels from the thyroid, oesophagus, heart and adrenals, the remainder traverse at least one and sometimes as many as 10 lymph nodes.

c F— Total lymph production is about 120 ml/hour (about 10 per cent of the capillary filtrate).

d T— Only a small proportion of filtered protein diffuses back to the venous capillaries.

326   The lymphatic vessels draining:

a   The stomach pass with the veins to the caval plexuses.   (   )

b   The tip of the tongue pass to the submental nodes.   (   )

c   The lower anal canal pass to the inguinal nodes.   (   )

d   The upper extremity differ from that of the lower extremity in that they follow the veins.   (   )

327   The lymph nodes:

a   Of the axilla number up to 20.   (   )

b   Of the parotid group drain the inner ear and external auditory meatus.   (   )

c   Of the left supraclavicular fossa are commonly implicated in gastrointestinal malignancy.   (   )

d   Are responsible for the production of plasma cells.   (   )

328   A cystic hygroma:

a   Is a lymphangioma.   (   )

b   Occurs most commonly in the second year of life.   (   )

c   Is usually situated in the posterior mediastinum.   (   )

d   Usually regresses at puberty.   (   )

329   Lymphoedema tarda:

a   Is a late complication of venous thrombosis.   (   )

b   Should be treated by varicose vein surgery.   (   )

c   Can be improved by postural drainage.   (   )

d   Should be treated with prophylactic antibiotics.   (   )

a   F— The gastric lymph vessels accompany the arteries (the regional nodes are named after them) before passing to the coeliac and superior mesenteric pre-aortic nodes.

b   T— The lateral aspect drains to submandibular nodes and the posterior third to retropharyngeal nodes.

c   T— But those of the upper anal canal pass to the inferior mesenteric nodes. This is an important factor in deciding the surgical approach to neoplasms of the anal canal.

d   F— The lymphatics of both upper and lower limbs follow the veins.

a   F— As many as 30 to 60 may be present, receiving the dermal lymphatics from the trunk and arm and also the majority of the breast tissue lymphatics.

b   T— The lymphatics draining the face also pass to this group. In malignant lesions of the face with nodal involvement a superficial parotidectomy may be necessary as the nodes are embedded in the gland.

c   T— This was observed by Virchow who was the first to link the lymphatic system with the spread of malignant disease.

d   T— These are involved in the production of humoral antibodies.

a   T— Which is usually congenital in origin.

b   F— The majority occur in the first year. 90 per cent have occurred before the end of the second year.

c   F— It is usually situated in the neck.

d   F— It may grow considerably during early childhood. Regression is very uncommon. Surgical cure is difficult but is indicated occasionally for cosmetic reasons or to relieve tracheal compression.

a   F— It is a primary lymphoedema of late onset.

b   F— Venous surgery should be avoided since any lymphatics that are present follow the veins and may be damaged.

c   T— Together with compression bandaging of the legs when the patient is ambulant.

d   F— Long term antibiotic therapy in lymphoedema is only necessary with frequently recurring attacks of cellulitis.

330   Secondary lymphoedema:

a   May be caused by *Wuchereria bancrofti.*   (   )

b   Of the arm in post-mastectomy patients undergoes   (   )
     lymphosarcomatous changes in 10 per cent of patients.

c   Is characterised by an increased number of lymphatics.   (   )

d   Is characterised by dermal backflow.   (ˎ)

331   In a lymphangiogram of the leg:

a   The contrast medium injected is water soluble.   (   )

b   The lymph vessel is first identified by injecting methylene   (   )
     blue into the webs of the toes or fingers.

c   The presence of 3 or 4 lymphatic channels ascending to the (   )
     inguinal nodes is normal.

d   The contrast medium must be injected within 5 minutes to   (   )
     give satisfactory X-rays.

332   The treatment of lymphangitis in a limb should include:

a   Active mobilisation to allow the muscle pump to maintain   (   )
     lymph flow.

b   Incision of any associated inflamed areas.   (   )

c   The use of an appropriate antibiotic.   (   )

d   Lymphangiography.   (   )

333   Acute arterial occlusion:

a   Should be treated conservatively if the site of the occlusion (   )
     is above the inguinal ligament.

b   Demands the urgent use of vasodilator drugs.   (   )

c   Of a limb is usually painless due to the anoxic damage   (   )
     produced in the peripheral nerves.

d   May produce irreversible muscle necrosis after 6 hours.   (   )

a **T**— The filarial larvae are transmitted by mosquitos. The adult worm lives primarily in the lymphatic vessels and nodes, causing lymphatic obstruction.

b **F**— This rare malignancy occurs in less than 0.5 per cent of such patients.

c **F**— The number of lymphatics is not increased but they are dilated.

d **T**— Demonstrating stasis and distension in the skin lymphatics.

a **F**— Ultrafluid lipiodol, a fat soluble contrast medium which remains in the lymphatics, is used.

b **T**— This outlines the dermal lymphatics which can then be entered with a fine cannula.

c **F**— Normally 10 or 12 channels are shown.

d **F**— The medium is dense and injection of the 8 ml required in under 10 minutes will rupture the lymph vessels.

a **F**— Rest and elevation reduce the lymph flow and help to localise infection.

b **F**— Only if an abscess is present is incision indicated.

c **T**— Lymphangitis indicates a failure of localisation of the infection and thus antibiotics should be used.

d **F**— This investigation has no place in the management of lymphangitis.

a **F**— Gangrene of the lower limbs frequently follows untreated saddle emboli and iliac vessel occlusion. Urgent surgical removal of the clot is thus indicated in the majority of patients.

b **F**— There are no pharmacological agents available which can improve on the vasodilatation that has already occurred in the ischaemic area.

c **F**— The pain is immediate and severe and worsens as muscle necrosis develops.

d **T**— The onset of this condition which soon becomes irreversible is indicated by the development of tenderness and spasm in the muscles together with muscle swelling. In such cases it may be necessary to decompress the muscular compartment by fasciotomy in addition to relieving the arterial obstruction.

334 In chronic arterial occlusion of the lower limbs:

a Buttock claudication is suggestive of arterial occlusion above the inguinal ligament.   ( )

b Skin ulceration most commonly occurs along the medial border of the foot.   ( )

c Which is severe, there may be venous 'guttering' on elevation of the legs.   ( )

d There is usually an associated peripheral neuropathy.   ( )

335 Abdominal aortic aneurysms:

a Arise from an atheromatous vessel in approximately 50 per cent of cases.   ( )

b Characteristically produce epigastric pain.   ( )

c Are associated with duodenal ulceration.   ( )

d Which are asymptomatic are relatively benign conditions and should not usually be resected.   ( )

336 Raynaud's disease:

a Is caused by an abnormal sensitivity of skin vessels to cold.   ( )

b Is marked by a characteristic pallor of the hands after cold stimulation followed by blue and then red colour changes.   ( )

c May be associated with scleroderma.   ( )

d Is permanently relieved by sympathectomy in the vast majority of cases.   ( )

a T— It is particularly common in internal iliac artery occlusion and therefore with severe disease of the common iliac arteries or the aorta.

b F— The commonest sites of skin ulceration are of the toes and in the interdigital clefts. Trauma frequently results in the heel or the lateral border of the foot becoming ulcerated.

c T— This, together with pallor on elevation and redness on dependency indicate a very inadequate arterial supply which is neither sufficient to produce venous filling nor to prevent anoxic vasodilation of the skin vessels.

d F— This is uncommon in uncomplicated chronic arterial obstruction. It does occur in diabetic patients with arterial disease and contributes to the high incidence of foot ulceration in these patients.

a F— Over 95 per cent of these aneurysms are atheromatous, the remainder are syphilitic, traumatic or mycotic in origin.

b F— The majority of aortic aneurysms are painless. However, when enlargement does occur, pain is felt in the flanks or in the back.

c T— There is an unexplained increase of duodenal ulceration in patients with aortic aneurysms and rupture may occur into the duodenum.

d F— Every patient with an aortic aneurysm, whether asymptomatic or not, is at risk of rupture, particularly when the aneurysm is larger than 7 cm or is tender. Only in relatively small aneurysms and in very aged or unfit patients is conservative management indicated.

a T— The disease has an unknown aetiology and is usually seen only in temperate zones. It is most common in young women appearing in the second and third decades.

b T— These changes are produced by intense and abnormal vasoconstriction which follows cold exposure and then after a period of several minutes' rewarming, an anoxic vasodilation of the skin vessels occurs. There is an initial sluggish and then a more rapid blood flow through the dilated and anoxic skin vessels.

c F— Collagen diseases, certain haematological disorders, occupational use of vibrating tools and sundry other unrelated diseases may be associated with Raynaud's phenomenon (see b above). Raynaud's disease however is the name given to the idiopathic disease defined in a.

d F— Less than three-quarters of the patients with Raynaud's disease are relieved by sympathectomy and of these in only half is the relief permanent.

337   **Common sites for atheromatous arterial aneurysms are:**
a   The femoral artery. ( )
b   The middle cerebral artery. ( )

c   The abdominal aorta. ( )

d   Intrarenal. ( )

338   **A dissecting aneurysm of the aorta:**
a   Usually starts around the aortic arch. ( )

b   Is so-called because of the extensive mediastinal destruction ( )
it produces when it ruptures.

c   Is associated with pregnancy. ( )
d   Is a feature of Marfan's syndrome. ( )

339   **Thromboangitis obliterans:**
a   Was originally described by a Japanese opthalmologist. ( )
b   Classically involves the branches of the aortic arch. ( )

c   Is a panarteritis. ( )

d   ·Is seen most frequently in young women. ( )

340   **The valves of the:**
a   Forearm communicating veins direct the flow from the deep ( )
to superficial veins.
b   The lower leg communicating veins direct the flow from ( )
the deep to superficial veins.

c   The thigh communicating veins direct the flow from the ( )
deep to superficial veins.
d   The upper arm communicating veins direct the flow from ( )
the deep to superficial veins.

a T— These are often bilateral and occur in association with aortic aneurysms.
b F— These are congenital and often produce symptoms before atheromatous changes have occurred, ie. between 20 and 30 years of age.
c T— This is the commonest site. The majority of aortic aneurysms lie below the renal vessels.
d F— When aneurysms occur intrarenally they are usually mycotic (i.e. infective in origin) and multiple.

a T— The commonest site of origin is just proximal or distal to the origin of the left subclavian artery.
b F— The dissection occurs in the arterial wall and is subintimal. When rupture occurs it is either retrogradely into the pericardium or distally close to the aortic bifurcation.
c T— There appears to be an increased incidence in young pregnant women.
d T— This is probably related to defective ground substance and decreased strength in the connective tissue of the arterial wall.

a F— It was first described by Buerger in 1909.
b F— It characteristically involves medium size arteries of the extremities such as the anterior and posterior tibial, radial and ulnar vessels.
c F— Histologically the major effects are found in the intima of the arteries and veins. It is not clear whether these are hypersensitivity phenomena or whether they are just the simple effects of thrombosis in a patient whose blood is 'hypercoagulable'.
d F— Thromboangitis obliterans is almost exclusively a disease in males. Cigarette smoking may have a part to play in the aetiology.
   (All statements in this question are true of Takayasu's disease—a very rare arteritis.)

a T— These veins perforate the deep fascia.

b F— In all these areas the valves of communicating veins allow blood to flow from superficial to deep veins where the 'muscle pump' forces the blood flow centrally.

c F

d F

341 **The long saphenous vein:**
a Arises on the medial aspect of the sole of the foot. ( )
b Passes 1 cm in front of the medial malleolus. ( )
c Passes behind the knee joint. ( )
d Enters the femoral sheath by piercing the fascia lata. ( )

342 **Commonly used sclerosants for varicose vein injection are:**
a 3 per cent sodium tetradecyl sulphate. ( )
b Thrombin. ( )
c Ethanolamine. ( )
d 5 per cent phenol in almond oil. ( )

343 **In deep venous thrombosis of the lower limb:**
a One of the most common sites of origin is the short saphenous vein. ( )
b One of the common sites of origin is in the iliofemoral segment. ( )
c The diagnosis can usually be made by clinical examination. ( )
d Tender swollen thrombosed veins are usually palpable. ( )

344 **The incidence of postoperative venous thrombosis can be reduced:**
a By raising the foot of the operating table during surgery. ( )
b By passive calf contractions during an operation. ( )
c By the intravenous administration of 500 ml of low molecular weight Dextran during operation and on the first two postoperative days. ( )
d By the prophylactic use of subcutaneous heparin. ( )

a F— It is a continuation of the medial end of the dorsal arch vein.
b T—
c T
d F— It passes through a defect in the fascia lata, the saphenous opening, to
        join the femoral vein.

a T— This detergent compound is used extensively in the technique of
        compression sclerotherapy for varicose veins.
b F— This could be lethal, giving rise to systemic coagulation effects.
c T— It is a less powerful sclerosant than a.
d F— This solution is used for paravenous injection of haemorrhoids.

a F— In the lower leg the soleal plexus is the usual site of origin of venous
        thrombosis.
b T— Iliofemoral thrombosis commonly follows hip or pelvic surgery and may
        also extend from the calf veins.
c F— There is almost no correlation between signs in the lower leg and the
        presence of deep vein thrombosis for many thrombi are non-occlusive
        and produce no ankle swelling or calf tenderness.
d F— These are the signs of superficial thrombophlebitis which is not usually
        related to deep vein thrombosis or associated with the risk of embolism.

a F— This is not of proven value.
b T— This reduces the risk of venous stasis.
c T— This is an effective prophylactic measure and acts by reducing blood
        viscosity and platelet aggregation.

d T— The administration of low doses of heparin in the preoperative and early
        postoperative period is effective in reducing the incidence of post-
        operative thrombosis.

345 **Venous ulcers of the lower limb:**

a Are usually the result of longstanding varicose veins.　( )

b Commonly follow deep venous thrombosis.　( )

c Most commonly occur below the medial malleolus.　( )

d Will usually heal when firm bandaging is applied.　( )

XVII Fractures and Dislocations

346 **A fracture is said to be:**

a Closed if an overlying skin laceration has been sutured.　( )

b Comminuted if there has been associated damage to adjacent nerves or vessels.　( )

c A fatigue fracture if it occurs through a diseased bone.　( )

d Pathological if it occurs through a bony metastasis.　( )

347 **In a healing fracture:**

a The haematoma is initially invaded by osteoblasts.　( )

b The tissue formed by the invading osteoblasts is termed osteoid.　( )

c Calcium salts are laid down in the osteoid tissue.　( )

d The final stage of repair is the remodelling of the callus.　( )

a F— Uncomplicated varicose veins even if present for many years do not usually produce ulcers, and when they do they are small and heal quickly.
b T— 'Venous' ulcers are nearly all postphlebitic in origin.
c F— The characteristic site is on the medial side of the ankle just above the malleolus.
d T— Bandaging provides continuous firm compression, preventing oedema and overcoming the increased pressure in the superficial veins of the postphlebitic limb.

a F— A closed fracture does not communicate with the exterior through a laceration or abrasion of the overlying skin or mucous membrane. Any fracture with an associated wound of the overlying skin or mucosa is said to be an open or compound fracture.
b F— Comminuted means that more than 2 fragments of bone are present. When there is a single fracture line, the fracture is described as simple, but if the broken ends are compressed into each other, the fracture is then said to be impacted.
c F— A fatigue fracture occurs in areas which undergo repeated stress, an example being the 'march' fracture of the 4th metatarsal which is usually sustained by healthy adults after an unaccustomed long walk.
d T— The term includes fractures through any diseased area of bone. Other examples include osteoporosis, osteogenesis imperfecta and Paget's disease.

a F— The haematoma is initially invaded by capillaries and fibroblasts. Calcium salts pass into solution in the acidic environment.
b T— Osteoblasts invade the healing wound at 10 to 14 days, the pH progressively becoming more alkaline. During this time the concentration of alkaline phosphatase in the wound tissues increases.
c T— This forms callus. The amount formed is to some extent related to the amount of stress on the fracture site, thus a fractured femur forms proportionately much more callus than a fractured metacarpal.
d T— The trabecular architecture of the bone becomes re-established and excess callus is then reabsorbed.

348   **Non-union is often seen in:**
a   Fractures of the 4th metatarsal.   (   )
b   Fractures of the neck of the femur.   (   )
c   Fractures of the condyle of the mandible.   (   )
d   Colles' fractures.   (   )

349   **Dislocation of the sternoclavicular joint:**
a   Is usually caused by a fall on the outstretched hand.   (   )

b   Displaces the clavicle upwards and medially.   (   )

c   Is usually treated by internal fixation.   (   )

d   Never causes any compression of the trachea or great vessels   (   )
    in the neck.

350   **Fractures of the clavicle:**
a   Are usually of the greenstick variety in children under the   (   )
    age of 10 years.
b   Are usually the result of direct violence.   (   )

c   Can be recognised by the abnormal elevation of the distal   (   )
    fragment.
d   Are usually treated by internal fixation.   (   )

351   **In fractures of the surgical neck of the humerus:**
a   The lesion is usually due to indirect violence.   (   )
b   The fragments are usually impacted.   (   )

c   The proximal fragment is usually internally rotated.   (   )

d   The distal fragment is usually adducted.   (   )

a   F—   Classical sites of non-union of fractures are the scaphoid, talus and the
b   T   neck of the femur. All the areas involved are relatively avascular.
c   F   Delayed union and non-union are more common in the aged, in those
d   F   fractures with associated infection, with inadequate fixation and when
              the bony ends are separated by excessive traction or by the interposition
              of soft tissues.

a   T—   This causes the medial end of the clavicle to rise anteriorly over the
              sternum.
b   T—   The weight of the arm and the pectoral muscles pull it medially while
              sternomastoid elevates the medial end of the clavicle.
c   T—   Reduction of both anterior and posterior dislocations can be achieved
              by bracing the shoulders. The attachments of the articular disc which
              give much of the strength to the joint will have been weakened and
              dislocation will re-occur unless some form of fixation is undertaken.
d   F—   Posterior dislocations may cause the medial end of the clavicle to impinge
              on the trachea and the great vessels in the neck. Operative reduction is
              then an urgent necessity.

a   T—   Thus displacement is minimal and treatment is usually only symptomatic.

b   F—   This fracture is usually due to falls on the outstretched palm. Direct
              trauma to the outer end usually leads to anterior buckling and injuries
              to the underlying subclavian vessels and brachial plexus are thus
              extremely uncommon.
c   F—   The proximal fragment is elevated by the sternomastoid but the distal
              fragment is depressed by the effect of gravity on the shoulder and arm.
d   F—   A figure-of-eight bandage provides some symptomatic relief and support.
              In most patients the fracture heals without internal fixation. The slight
              deformity presents few problems.

a   T—   The most frequent cause being a fall on the outstretched hand.
b   T—   Although the fracture is frequently comminuted, the bone in this
              region is very cancellous and impacts easily.
c   F—   The rotator cuff muscles are both internal and external rotators of the
              shoulder. Supinator acts on the proximal fragment producing abduction.
d   T—   The overall displacement is not usually extensive and is accepted. Early
              mobilisation is encouraged.

352 **In a fracture of the distal third of the shaft of the humerus:**

a   The distal fragment is usually posteriorly angulated by the   (   )
action of biceps.

b   The radial nerve is frequently damaged.   (   )

c   Delayed radial nerve palsy is usually due to oedema.   (   )

d   Late onset of radial nerve palsy is usually due the involve-   (   )
ment of the nerve with callus.

353 **A supracondylar fracture of the humerus:**

a   Is a fracture commonly seen in young adults.   (   )

b   Is particularly subject to the complication of ischaemic   (   )
muscle contracture.

c   Is held in the position of reduction by the tendon of   (   )
brachioradialis.

d   When properly reduced has the index finger pointing   (   )
approximately to the tip of the shoulder of the same side.

354 **A transverse fracture of the scaphoid is:**

a   Prone to infection.   (   )
b   Usually seen in young men.   (   )

c   Prone to avascular necrosis.   (   )

d   Usually seen on an early scaphoid X-ray.   (   )

a F— The elbow is usually held flexed, relaxing biceps, and any angulation is
       then anterior due to triceps contraction. In proximal fractures of the
       shaft of the humerus deltoid and pectoralis major muscles both act on
       the proximal fragment to produce considerable angulation.
b T— The radial nerve lies close to the bone in the radial groove and can thus
       be easily damaged with fracture at this site.
c F— If a delayed radial nerve palsy appears, it is almost certainly due to
       movement and trauma from a sharp fracture surface.
d T— If this is the case, then operative treatment and neurolysis (removal of
       the nerve from the proximity of the healing fracture) may be necessary.

a F— This is usually a fracture of childhood; and frequently follows a fall on
       the outstretched hand with the elbow flexed.
b T— The brachial artery is frequently traumatised in this lesion and may be
       lacerated or put into spasm. When this occurs the muscles of the forearm
       may undergo ischaemic necrosis and contracture.
c F— The triceps muscle posteriorly and the brachialis muscle anteriorly are
       the closest and most powerful relations of this part of the humerus and
       they have a splinting effect on the reduced fracture.
d T— And reduction is keyed by traction on the distal fragment followed by
       flexion at the elbow. Care must be taken at all times to ensure that the
       radial pulse is present. It is essential to cut out a window in the plaster at
       the wrist so that the radial artery can be frequently checked.

a F— It is rarely compound so infection is not a problem.
b T— This injury is sustained by falling on the outstretched hand. In older
       patients this same injury produces a Colles' fracture.
c T— Prolonged immobilisation minimises the risk of avascular necrosis and
       non-union. For this reason plasters are worn until radiological healing is
       present.
d F— Fractures of the scaphoid are often not seen on the earliest X-rays and
       the diagnosis must be made clinically (a painful wrist with tenderness in
       the anatomical snuff box). Reduction is best achieved with the wrist
       flexed. Repeat X-rays taken two weeks after the injury may then
       demonstrate some local reabsorption of bone around the fracture and
       thus render it more obvious.

355 **In a Colles' fracture the distal radial fragment:**
a   Is dorsally angulated on the proximal radius. ( )

b   Is usually torn from the intra-articular triangular disc. ( )

c   Is deviated to the ulnar side. ( )
d   Is usually impacted. ( )

356 **In a Monteggia fracture dislocation:**
a   The dislocation of the distal radio-ulnar joint brings the ( )
    ulnar styloid process anterior to the capitulum.
b   The radial fracture is usually at the junction of the middle ( )
    and distal thirds.
c   Internal fixation is usually required in the adult. ( )
d   The causative injury is often a blow on the extensor surface ( )
    of the forearm with the elbow flexed.

357 **Dislocations of the shoulder joint:**
a   Most commonly occur in middle age. ( )
b   Usually occur when the arm is in the abducted position. ( )

c   Usually have the head of the humerus situated behind the ( )
    glenoid fossa.
d   Are often recurrent in the young. ( )

358 **Fractures of the maxilla:**
a   Cannot usually be demonstrated radiologically for 48 hours. ( )

b   Are often accompanied by numbness over the upper lip. ( )

c   Are often accompanied by diplopia. ( )

d   Rarely require surgical intervention. ( )

a   T— It is also dorsally displaced to produce the typical 'dinner fork' abnormality.

b   F— The ulna styloid (to which the disc is also attached) is often avulsed but the intra-articular disc of fibrocartilage is far too strong to be torn.

c   F— The distal radial fragment is always radially deviated.

d   T— Therefore reduction of a Colles' fracture should include traction (to overcome impaction), flexion (to overcome dorsal angulation) and ulnar deviation (to overcome radial deviation).

a   F— The dislocation is of the head of the radius from the superior radio-ulnar joint.

b   F— The radius is not fractured. The fracture is in the shaft of the ulnar at the junction of the proximal and middle thirds.

c   T— Though in a child the reduction is generally stable.

d   T— Though it is probably more frequently produced by a fall on the outstretched hand.

a   F— They are commonest in young adults who indulge in athletic pursuits.

b   T— The shoulder joint is at its most unstable in this position and may dislocate with a trivial blow.

c   F— The head of the humerus is usually displaced anteriorly.

d   T— Dislocation of the shoulder joint tends to produce laxity in the capsule of the joint and the joint is subsequently less stable.

a   F— If suitable views are taken the fracture lines will be seen immediately and there will be opacity of the appropriate maxillary sinus.

b   T— The infraorbital nerve is usually damaged as the fracture line typically passes through the infraorbital canal.

c   T— The fracture may involve the bony attachments of the suspensory ligament of the eye.

d   F— Some form of fixation is usually necessary to avoid persistent diplopia, limitation of jaw movement and cosmetic deformity.

359 **In pelvic fractures:**

a Avulsion injuries are usually treated by early mobilisation. ( )

b Undisplaced lesions of the ischial or pubic rami are usually ( )
treated by early mobilisation.

c Extraperitoneal urinary extravasation may be due to damage ( )
either to the membraneous urethra or to the base of the
bladder.

d Which are unstable, one half of the pelvis is displaced ( )
proximally by the flank muscles. Reduction may need 40
to 50 lb (18 to 23 kg) of traction.

360 **Intracapsular fractures of the upper end of the femur are
usually:**

a Accompanied by shortening of the leg. ( )

b Accompanied by external rotation of the leg. ( )
c Accompanied by adduction of the leg. ( )

d Treated by internal fixation. ( )

361 **Extracapsular fractures of the upper end of the femur are
usually:**

a Subtrochanteric in position. ( )

b Subject to avascular necrosis of the head of the femur. ( )

c Accompanied by internal rotation of the leg. ( )

d Treated by internal fixation. ( )

a **T—** These injuries affect the anterior superior and inferior iliac spines and are the result of violent muscle contractions. They do not effect the stability of the pelvis and thus do not require prolonged immobilisation.

b **T—** These injuries are usually due to direct trauma. The stability of the pelvis is not markedly affected and weight bearing can be resumed once the initial pain has subsided.

c **T—** Rupture of the puboprostatic ligament may be associated with tearing of the prostate from the membranous urethra. Bony fragments of the fractured pubis may pierce the bladder.

d **T—** In addition severe pelvic fractures are accompanied by extensive haemorrhage (often concealed), shock and possible bladder and rectal injuries.

a **T—** This is the result of the longitudinal pull of the hamstring, rectus femoris and iliopsoas muscles.

b **T—** This is due to the action of iliopsoas acting distal to the fracture.

c **F—** Adductor and abductor muscles are both attached to the distal shaft and their actions are thus counterbalanced.

d **T—** This reduces the incidence of avascular necrosis and subsequent non-union. Internal fixation also speeds up mobilisation in these patients who are commonly quite elderly. Very occasionally undisplaced impacted fractures are treated non-surgically.

a **F—** The fracture most commonly lies between the greater and lesser trochanters, i.e. is an intertrochanteric fracture.

b **F—** In this type of fracture healing is usually uneventful. The major part of the blood supply to the head of the femur comes through capsular vessels which are usually undamaged in extracapsular fractures.

c **F—** These fractures show shortening and external rotation as in the intracapsular variety. In addition adduction of the leg is present as the adductor muscles act on the distal fragment without the opposition of the glutei which remain attached to the proximal fragment.

d **T—** The most commonly used prostheses include a long plate which is screwed onto the upper femoral shaft and a pin which is inserted into the proximal fragment.

362   In fractures of the mid shaft of the femur:

a   The proximal fragment is usually flexed.   (   )

b   The proximal fragment is usually abducted.   (   )

c   The distal fragment is usually adducted.   (   )

d   The common femoral vessels are usually damaged.   (   )

363   In fractures of the patella:

a   Comminution is usual when the fracture has been caused by   (   )
       indirect violence.

b   A transverse fracture without displacement is usually   (   )
       treated by a plaster cylinder with no direct surgical
       intervention.

c   A comminuted fracture is best treated by patella excision and   (   )
       replacement by a prosthesis.

d   Weight bearing should be avoided for the first week.   (   )

364   In fractures of the middle third of the tibia and fibula:

a   Delayed union is common.   (   )

b   Indirect violence usually results in a spiral or oblique   (   )
       fracture line.

c   Shortening and anterior angulation of the tibia are common.   (   )

d   Comminuted fractures are usually treated by early   (   )
       plating of the tibia.

a T— Since the hip flexors are unopposed by the effect of gravity on the distal leg.

b T— The attachment of the glutei muscles to the greater trochanter achieves this and the proximal fragment is usually externally rotated.

c T— This is due to the unopposed action of the adductor muscles. The hamstrings and quadriceps also produce some shortening of the leg.

d F— Extensive bleeding may occur particularly from the profunda vessels but the main artery and vein are not usually directly involved.

a F— Transverse fractures are more common in this fracture usually produced by acute flexion of the knee. Direct injuries to the patella usually produce comminuted fractures.

b T— The fragments may be held together by the capsule of the knee joint, although there is frequently a large haemarthrosis present which will require aspiration.

c F— Excision is only advisable in very severely comminuted fractures and even if this is necessary no prosthesis is required. Tendon suture provides quite good knee flexion.

d F— Provided the knee is maintained in extension, weight bearing can be readily undertaken. Active quadriceps exercise may be started on about the 10th day after the injury.

a T— These fractures are frequently compound. There is a relatively poor blood supply to the bones in this region, and interposition of muscle and superadded infection are frequent complications. Therefore the incidence of delayed union is high.

b T— Particularly if a twisting force is imparted to the foot.

c T— The anterior surface of the tibia is unsupported by muscles and no splinting effect occurs.

d F— These fractures are usually due to direct injury and are compound. Internal fixation is therefore best avoided.

365   **In injuries of the ankle joint:**
a   Eversion injuries are the most commonly encountered.   ( )
b   Inversion injuries are usually accompanied by a tear of the deltoid ligament.   ( )
c   There is frequently associated posterior tibial nerve damage.   ( )
d   The joint is rendered unstable by rupture of the inferior tibio-fibular ligament.   ( )

366   **Dislocation of the hip joint:**
a   Is most common when the hip is in a neutral position.   ( )
b   Is usually associated with a fracture of the acetabular rim.   ( )
c   Usually results in the femoral head coming to lie anteriorly over the pubis or obturator externus.   ( )
d   May be associated with injuries of the sciatic nerve.   ( )

367   **In spinal fractures:**
a   The odontoid process is usually damaged by extension injuries.   ( )
b   Of the base of the odontoid process, the odontoid process is carried forward with the atlas.   ( )
c   Non-union of the odontoid is uncommon.   ( )
d   Involving a spinous process treatment is usually by internal fixation.   ( )

XVIII   Orthopaedic Surgery

368   **In rheumatoid arthritis:**
a   The principal lesion is an area of fibrinoid necrosis surrounded by fibroblasts.   ( )
b   The synovial membrane characteristically undergoes marked hypertrophy.   ( )
c   The fibrosis in the joint capsule and ligaments produces the main deforming forces in the early stages of the disease.   ( )
d   The permanent deformity in the late stage of the disease is usually due to bone ankylosis.   ( )

a   F— The ankle is more unstable in the inverted position.
b   F— This injury affects the lateral not the medial ligament of the joint.

c   F— Nerve and vascular complications are exceedingly rare.

d   T— This injury requires external or internal fixation for six weeks prior to any weight bearing.

a   F— The most common dislocation is a posterior one and this is usually the result of force along the line of the femoral shaft when it is flexed at a right angle as in the sitting position. Thus, motorcyclists suffering a sudden deceleration frequently sustain posterior dislocations of the hip.
b   T— The posterior margin of the rim is most commonly affected.
c   F— This form of dislocation is occasionally seen but in the common posterior dislocation the head lies posterior to the acetabulum.
d   T— This serious, and sometimes permanent, disability sometimes complicates posterior dislocation of the hip.

a   F— The commonest causes are flexion injuries such as occur in violent deceleration or from a blow to the back of the head.
b   T— It is maintained in this position by the transverse ligaments of the atlas.

c   F— The initial fracture may be painless and difficult to demonstrate but late films will show an area of sclerosis.
d   F— These, like fractures of a transverse process, are usually avulsion injuries and require no specific surgery. Active mobilisation should be encouraged once the initial pain has subsided.

a   T— These are the characteristic changes of the rheumatoid nodule.

b   T— This feature accounts for the joint swelling and the inflammatory mass which extends over the articular surface (known as the pannus).
c   F— The early deformity is due to the laxity of the diseased capsule and ligaments together with associated muscle spasm.
d   F— Although bone ankylosis does occur it is rare. These permanent deformities are usually due to peri-articular fibrosis.

369   Rheumatoid arthritis:

a   Is characteristically symmetrical in its involvement of the   (   )
more proximal joints.

b   Has an equivalent disease in childhood which is also   (   )
associated with pericarditis.

c   Carries a worse prognosis if serological tests (such as the   (   )
Rose Waller and Latex tests) are positive.

d   Is characterised by the pes anserinus deformity.   (   )

370   Acute osteomyelitis in childhood:

a   Is usually the result of compound bony injuries.   (   )

b   Is characterised by a constant bone pain.   (   )

c   Characteristically produces necrosis of the periosteum   (   )
overlying the infected bone.

d   Is not demonstrable radiologically for the first 2 weeks of   (   )
the disease.

371   In tuberculosis of the bone:

a   The local reaction is characterised by extensive new bone   (   )
formation.

b   The metaphysis of a long bone is the commonest site of   (   )
involvement.

c   The infection is usually secondary to a primary focus   (   )
elsewhere in the body.

d   Extension of the bone abscess into a joint is common.   (   )

a   **T—** The disease starts distally and gradually extends to more proximal joints.

b   **T—** Still's disease—the childhood equivalent—is also characterised by skin rashes, lymphadenopathy and splenomegaly. The illness usually produces more systemic effects and is more rapid in onset than the adult form.

c   **T—** These tests are positive in approximately 25 per cent of cases.

d   **F—** This term has no connection with rheumatoid arthritis (it in fact describes the division of the facial nerve). The proximal interphalangeal joints frequently show however a swan neck deformity produced by hyperextension of these joints.

a   **F—** It is usually haematogenous in origin, arising from foci such as boils, infected tonsils or urinary tract infections. Exogenous infections are more common in the adult form of the disease.

b   **T—** A constant pain of increasing severity is present from the earliest stages of the infection.

c   **F—** Bone necrosis frequently follows acute osteomyelitis. The dead bone is known as a sequestrum. The overlying periosteum usually survives and forms new subperiosteal bone known as the involucrum which thus often surrounds a subperiosteal abscess.

d   **T—** Radiological evidence of bone infection may not be evident until the first subperiosteal new bone appears in 14 to 21 days. Antibiotic treatment must be instituted on clinical grounds as soon as the diagnosis is made.

a   **F—** In bone tuberculosis, osteoporosis and bone lysis is usually present. There is much less tendency to new bone formation than in pyogenic bone infection.

b   **F—** The infection nearly always starts in the epiphysis.

c   **T—** It is a blood-borne metastatic infection which spreads from primary foci in the lungs, bowel or lymph nodes.

d   **T—** This is a consequence of the location of the infection and often results in joint destruction and extension of the abscess into the surrounding soft tissues. The abscesses show few of the classical signs of inflammation and may grow to a large size before presentation.

372   **In osteoarthritis of the hip joint:**

a   The articular cartilage undergoes initial hypertrophy and   ( )
then becomes hardened and eburnated.

b   The joint capsule becomes stretched and lax.   ( )

c   The leg is usually adducted and externally rotated when the   ( )
patient lies supine.

d   A femoral osteotomy usually helps halt the progress of the   ( )
disease process.

373   **In Paget's disease of the bone:**

a   The serum alkaline phosphatase is considerably raised.   ( )

b   Spiral fractures of the femur are common.   ( )

c   Deafness is a characteristic of the later stages of the disease.   ( )

d   Osteogenic sarcoma develops twice as commonly as in   ( )
unaffected people.

374   **Dyschondroplasia is characterised by:**

a   A large skull with a short base and a snub nose.   ( )

b   Short stubby fingers (the trident hand).   ( )

c   Being inherited as a Mendelian dominant.   ( )

d   Multiple enchondromata of the fingers and toes.   ( )

375   **Diaphysial aclasis is characterised by:**

a   A defect in cartilagenous ossification.   ( )

b   Multiple fractures and subsequent deformity.   ( )

c   Blue sclera.   ( )

d   Being familial in origin.   ( )

a   F— The articular cartilage thins and becomes rough; the underlying bone
then becomes dense and smooth (eburnated) and cysts usually develop
in the perichondral bone.

b   F— The capsule becomes thick and fibrosed. At the extremes of movement
some tearing may occur and this gives rise to further fibrosis.

c   T— Some degree of fixed flexion deformity is also commonly present.

d   T— In some cases the joint changes are partly reversed. The operation should
be performed before the head of the femur has collapsed. Improvement
is unlikely if this has already occurred.

a   T

b   F— Though pathological fractures of the femur do occur in this condition,
they are usually of the transverse variety and are typically in the
subtrochanteric region of the femur.

c   T— The bony thickening and deformity commonly involves the skull and
may thus interfere with the transmission of sound vibrations. The spine,
femur and tibia are the commonest sites of involvement.

d   F— There is a greatly increased rate of osteogenic sarcoma formation in these
patients. It is more than 30 times that of the normal population and the
tumour appears to be a particularly malignant variety.

a   F— These are all features of achondroplasia—typified by the short limbed

b   F   circus dwarf. There is frequently a lordosis present.

c   F

d   T— The disease is also known as multiple enchondromatosis or Ollier's
disease. It is due to the failure of ossification of areas of cartilage in the
epiphyses. It is not familial.

a   T— The condition is also known as multiple exostosis. Large bony outgrowths
appear at the ends of long bones arising from the epiphyseal plate.

b   F— These features are typical of osteogenesis imperfecta which often presents

c   F   with frequent fractures following trivial trauma at birth (as a stillbirth)
or in later childhood (osteogenesis imperfecta tarda).

d   T— And it is commoner in males.

376 **Dupuytren's contracture of the palm:**
a Is transmitted as a Mendelian dominant. (　)
b Is predominantly seen in men. (　)
c Has an association with glomerulonephritis. (　)
d Which is longstanding, is often associated with secondary (　)
   fibrosis of the interphalangeal joints.

377 **In a case of congenital dislocation of the hip:**
a There is a defect of the posterior rim of the acetabulum. (　)

b On bilateral hip abduction with the knees flexed there is often (　)
   limited abduction on the diseased side.
c Reduction is sometimes hindered by a tight gluteus (　)
   minimus muscle.

d Splinting of the limbs following reduction should be (　)
   maintained until the femoral epiphysis returns to its normal
   density on X-ray examination.

378 **Slipped femoral epiphyses:**
a Occur between the ages of 5 and 10 years. (　)
b Typically are seen in overweight children. (　)
c Are bilateral in 20 per cent of patients. (　)
d Are displaced downwards and posterior in relation to the (　)
   neck of the femur.

379 **Perthes disease of the hip:**
a Is a degenerative disease of the elderly. (　)

b Often presents with a fixed flexion deformity of the hip. (　)

c May, in most cases, be treated non-surgically. (　)

d Has a better prognosis when diagnosed in a younger patient. (　)

a   **F—** There is, however, an inherited predisposition to this disease.
b   **T—** The frequency is 10 : 1.
c   **F—** It is associated with liver disease and chronic alcoholism.
d   **T—** This may necessitate amputation of the digit.

a   **F—** The acetabular defect is superior, although the dislocation is always posterior. The consistency of this defect is one of the factors supporting the genetic theory of origin (20 per cent familial). Other theories are abnormal intrauterine positioning and capsular laxity due to maternal hormones.
b   **T—** This is the basis of Ortolani's test—the hip often clicking (or jerking) into position to allow further abduction.
c   **F—** Characteristic causes limiting a closed reduction are a tight psoas muscle, an hour glass stricture of the capsule, a thick ligamentum teres and an infolding of the superior labrum glenoidale (known as the limbus).
d   **F—** Reduction should be maintained until the acetabular roof re-forms, which takes 6 to 9 months in those cases diagnosed early.

a   **F—** The age of peak incidence is 10 to 15 years.
b   **T—** Boys are affected more commonly than girls.
c   **T—** Careful follow-up is therefore essential.
d   **T—** A lateral X-ray is therefore the most informative.

a   **F—** This is a disease of young children particularly between the ages of 5 and 10 years. Boys are affected four times more frequently than girls. It is thought to be due to an ischaemic necrosis of the epiphysis of the head of the femur.
b   **F—** The usual presentation is with pain in the hip and a limp. X-rays may show fragmentation, flattening and increased density of the femoral head.
c   **T—** The deformity of the femoral head and thus the long-term sequelae are minimised by non-weight-bearing (often for more than one year).
d   **T—** This is probably due to the smaller epiphysis in the young child which has a better chance of being revascularised.

380 **Idiopathic scoliosis:**
a Is the most common type of scoliosis. ( )

b Usually appears between the ages of 10 and 12 years. ( )

c Is more common in boys. ( )
d Is sometimes familial. ( )

381 **In benign tumours of cartilage:**
a Chondromata and osteochondromata occur equally in the ( )
two sexes.
b Malignant changes occur in 10 per cent of cases of multiple ( )
osteochondromata.
c Chondromata usually occur in the epiphyses of long bones. ( )

d Osteochondromata usually occur in the epiphyses of long ( )
bones.

382 **Chordomata:**
a Of the base of the skull (spheno-occipital) develop in the ( )
remnants of Rathke's pouch.
b Of the sacrococcygial region develop in the remnants of the ( )
neural canal.
c Are characterised radiologically by central rarefaction of ( )
the bone and cortical thinning and expansion.
d Are commoner in females than in males. ( )

383 **An osteoid osteoma:**
a Usually presents in the adult. ( )
b Is most frequently seen in the bones of the upper limb. ( )

c Commonly presents with local pain. ( )
d Demonstrates a small circular band of bony sclerosis ( )
surrounding a translucent area on X-rays.

a   **T—**   The scoliotic deformity produced is severe in this group (the worst being due to the paralytic form).

b   **T—**   There often is marked deterioration over the following years until the completion of vertebral growth.

c   **F—**   There is a predominance of this condition in girls. It has been suggested

d   **T**   that the condition is due to subclinical poliomyelitis but as the latter is equally distributed in both sexes this appears unlikely. The familial tendency may indicate a genetic aetiology.

a   **T—**   But the benign chondroblastoma is commoner in males.

b   **T—**   But this is less common in solitary tumours and occurs rarely in chondroblastomata.

c   **F—**   These tumours are usually present in the metaphysis of long bones, particularly in the bones of the hands and feet.

d   **F—**   These tumours are usually seen in the metaphysis of long bones. Chondroblastomata occur primarily in the epiphyses.

a   **F—**   These tumours develop from notochordal remnants and usually occur at its cephalic or caudal extremity.

b   **F**

c   **F—**   The characteristic radiological appearances are progressive bone destruction and soft tissue swelling.

d   **F—**   They are twice as common in males and present usually after the age of 30. The symptoms are mainly due to neural involvement.

a   **F—**   It most commonly presents during adolescence.

b   **F—**   Any bone may be involved but there is a slight predilection for the bones of the lower limb.

c   **T—**   Particularly so at night. Local tenderness also occurs.

d   **T—**   These are the characteristic radiographic appearances of osteoid osteoma and they may be confused with those of a chronic pyogenic bone abscess.

384   The osteoclastoma (giant cell tumour of bone):

a   Characteristically occurs in the shaft of a long bone.   (   )

b   Is more common in females than males.   (   )

c   May be recognised by the subperiosteal new bone which overlies the tumour and is demonstrable radiologically.

d   Is very rarely malignant.   (   )

385   Osteogenic sarcomata:

a   Are most frequent in the 10 to 25 year age group.   (   )

b   Readily metastasise via the blood stream.   (   )

c   Are frequently surrounded by non-malignant new bone formation.   (   )

d   When treated by conventional methods have a 50 per cent 5 year survival rate.   (   )

386   The Ewing's sarcoma of bone:

a   Is classically a disease of middle age and late years.   (   )

b   Can be effectively treated by radiotherapy.   (   )

c   Frequently results in a pathological fracture.   (   )

d   Usually occurs in the metaphyses of the long bones.   (   )

a   F—   It is almost invariably situated at the end of a bone. It can occur in any bone but is rare in flat bones.

b   F—   It is twice as common in males and the commonest age of presentation is in the third and fourth decades.

c   F—   Radiological characteristics do not include subperiosteal new bone. There is cortical expansion and thinning, together with rarefaction of the underlying bone. The cortex may be totally destroyed in the later stages of the disease.

d   F—   Local recurrence is present in almost half the cases after attempted surgical removal and malignant change is seen in about 15 per cent. Treatment should be by wide excision.

a   T—   The majority occur in this age group, exceptions being those occurring in late life in patients with Paget's disease of the bone. Common sites are around the knee and shoulder joint.

b   T—   Pulmonary metastases are particularly common. Lymph node metastases are very uncommon.

c   T—   The periosteum overlying an osteogenic sarcoma is raised by the tumour. This produces the characteristic radiological appearances of the overlying periosteum having underneath it a triangular area of new bone formation (Codman's triangle). The tumour itself comprises radiating spicules of new bone formation ('sunray') and variable degrees of lysis and sclerosis.

d   F—   Radical surgery is usually combined with preoperative radiotherapy. Not more than 5 to 10 per cent of patients survive 5 years. Recently there have been encouraging reports of improved survival figures after the use of multiple chemotherapy.

a   F—   The usual presentation is in infancy and up to the age of 25. It is more frequent in males.

b   F—   Survival varies from a few months to a few years. Whilst radiotherapy provides some symptomatic relief, neither this nor surgery is usually curative. The tumour is often multicentric in origin.

c   F—   The most frequent radiographic appearance is of overlapping layers of new subperiosteal bone formation, the so called 'onion peel' effect. This new bone has normal strength, thus pathological fractures are very uncommon.

d   T—   It is extremely uncommon for any other portion of the bone or any other type of bone to be affected.

387 Fibrosarcomata of the bone:

a   Are the most malignant of bone tumours.   (   )

b   Most commonly occur in the bones of the tarsus.   (   )

c   Demonstrate bone destruction with no new bone formation   (   )
     on X-ray.

d   Usually present with pulmonary metastases.   (   )

388 Chondrosarcomata:

a   Which develop in the metaphysis are usually less well   (   )
     differentiated than those occurring around the epiphysis.

b   Quite commonly invade the neighbouring blood vessels.   (   )

c   Commonly metastasise to lymph nodes.   (   )

d   Characteristically present as a pathological fracture.   (   )

XIX Neurosurgery

389 Intracranial aneurysms:

a   Are the cause of the vast majority of cases of spontaneous   (   )
     subarachnoid haemorrhage.

b   Are multiple in 20 per cent of cases.   (   )

c   Frequently rebleed after an initial haemorrhage.   (   )

d   Which have ruptured require surgical treatment which involves   (   )
     clipping of the appropriate middle cerebral artery.

a F— They are slower growing than osteogenic sarcomata and a five year
      survival rate of approximately 25 per cent is frequently reported.
      Treatment is by radical amputation.
b F— The sites of predilection are similar to those of the osteogenic sarcoma,
      i.e. in the ends of long bones, particularly the femur, tibia and humerus.
c T— The absence of radiating bone spiculation distinguishes it from osteogenic
      sarcoma.
d F— The most usual presentation is of a local, painful, progressive swelling
      around the knee, elbow or shoulder joint and sometimes a pathological
      fracture.

a T— Metaphyseal tumours often develop from osteochondromata whereas the
      peripheral tumours are formed of more mature cartilage. These tumours
      are slightly commoner in males and occur between the ages of 30 and 60
      years.
b T— Extension into the blood vessels is quite frequent.
c F— Metastases are usually seen late in the disease and are blood-borne,
      commonly producing peripheral lung deposits. Lymph node metastases
      are rare.
d F— The commonest presentation is of a painful bony swelling. Tenderness
      is present, particularly when haemorrhage and extraosseous extension has
      occurred.

a F— Intracranial aneurysms are the cause of over 50 per cent of spontaneous
      subarachnoid haemorrhage but the remainder are due to arteriovenous
      malformations, blood dyscrasias, antiocoagulant therapy and hyper-
      tension, together with a large group of unknown aetiology.
b T— These occur at arterial bifurcations around the circle of Willis.
c T— This carries with it a higher morbidity and mortality than the first bleed.
d F— Surgical treatment where indicated is directed at (i) excluding the
      aneurysm by clipping it at its neck, (ii) reinforcing its walls with fascia or
      synthetic material, or (iii) promoting thrombosis by injecting into it or
      by reducing its blood flow, e.g. by a carotid ligation. Clipping of the
      middle cerebral artery will usually produce serious neurological
      complications.

390   **In head injuries the causes of a rising intracranial pressure**
       include:
a   Intracerebral haemorrhage.   (   )

b   Cerebral oedema.   (   )

c   Rhinorrhoea.   (   )

d   Meningitis.   (   )

391   **In head injuries the signs of an expanding intracranial lesion**
       include:
a   A falling level of consciousness.   (   )

b   A rising pulse rate.   (   )
c   A falling blood pressure.   (   )

d   Small pupils.   (   )

392   **Following head injuries surgical intervention is usually**
       required for:
a   Linear skull fractures.   (   )
b   Cerebral oedema.   (   )

c   Depressed skull fractures.   (   )
d   Extradural haemorrhage.   (   )

a T— This is one of the three common types of post-traumatic intracranial haemorrhage. The others are considered in subsequent questions.

b T— This may develop within a few hours and contribute to the mortality of severe cases. It is normally treated by diuretic therapy and fluid restriction. Some success has been reported following administration of steroids.

c F— This and ottorrhoea usually subside within a few days. If they persist, craniotomy and some form of surgical repair of the dura is undertaken. It is not directly related to increasing intracranial pressure.

d T— This may follow closed as well as open cerebral injuries but is it more common in the latter. Prophylactic antibacterial therapy is indicated in open injuries.

a T— This is the most important of signs. Ensure that reproducible factors (such as whether or not the patient knows his name, age and address and the manner in which he obeys simple commands) are fully recorded at frequent intervals.

b F— The reverse is the case, the pulse rate falls and the blood pressure rises.

c F These vital signs must be observed at least every 15 minutes until normal stable values are maintained.

d F— These may be present in the initial stage due to stimulation of the oculomotor nerve but progressive increase in pressure shifts the brain and puts pressure on the oculomotor nerves resulting in pupillary dilatation (small pupils are seen with pontine injuries and these carry a very bad prognosis).

a F— Linear skull fractures demand careful observation of the patient's vital

b F signs in order to detect such complications as haemorrhage or infection. In the absence of these signs they do not require surgery. There is no satisfactory surgical cure for post-traumatic cerebral oedema.

c T— Surgery is required in all but minor depressions over non-vital areas.

d T— This is usually due to damage of the middle meningeal vessels often in association with linear fractures of the temporal bone. Typically the patient loses consciousness at the time of the accident due to concussion. Consciousness then returns (the so called lucid interval) until increasing intracranial pressure results in a falling of the level of consciousness. Emergency surgery is indicated to evacuate the clot and control the haemorrhage.

393   Chronic subdural haematomata:

a   Are common in the young.   (   )

b   Have a characteristic angiographic appearance.   (   )

c   Should be treated surgically.   (   )
d   Have a better postoperative prognosis than acute subdural   (   )
      haematomata.

**394   The characteristic signs of chronically raised intracranial pressure
       include:**

a   A bitemporal hemianopia.   (   )

b   Papilloedema.   (   )

c   Epilepsy.   (   )
d   Bradycardia.   (   )

395   In a patient with a lumbar disc protrusion:

a   Loss of the knee jerk is characteristic of a second lumbar   (   )
      nerve root lesion.
b   Loss of dorsiflexion of the great toes indicates a third   (   )
      lumbar nerve root lesion.
c   Loss of sensation over the sole indicates a fourth lumbar   (   )
      nerve root lesion.
d   Loss of the ankle jerk indicates a first sacral root lesion.   (   )

**396   In lesions affecting the common peroneal (lateral popliteal)
       nerve:**

a   Sensory loss is limited to the dorsal aspect of the first   (   )
      interdigital cleft.

b   There is weakness of dorsiflexion of the foot.   (   )
c   There is weakness of eversion of the foot.   (   )
d   The toes become clawed.   (   )

a **F—** They occur characteristically in the aged and often follow quite minor injuries. They are rarely associated with skull fractures.

b **T—** The cortical vessels are displaced from the vault and there is a shift in the midline structures away from the side of the lesion.

c **T—** Acute subdural haemorrhage follows severe trauma and is often bilateral.

d **T** It is associated with more severe underlying permanent damage to the brain, and has a worse prognosis than the chronic subdural haematomata. The latter should be treated surgically since they are generally associated with very minor underlying cerebral injury and the results are good.

a **F—** This characteristically follows pressure on the optic decussation from a pituitary tumour or a suprasellar meningioma.

b **T—** Papilloedema accompanies a raised intracranial pressure and is not, in its early phase, accompanied by visual symptoms.

c **T—** This may be grand mal or focal in nature.

d **T—** This is probably caused by the effect of pressure on the vasomotor centre. Other signs include a falling conscious level and a sixth nerve palsy.

a **F—** The knee jerk is mediated via the third and fourth lumbar nerve roots.

b **F—** This useful physical sign indicates a lesion of the fifth lumbar nerve root.

c **F—** The sole is supplied via the first sacral nerve root.

d **T**

a **F—** This is the area of sensory loss associated with lesions of the anterior tibial nerve. Involvement of the common peroneal nerve gives rise to sensory loss over the lateral aspect of the leg and the dorsum of the foot.

b **T—** The patient suffers from foot drop and walks with a high stepping gait on

c **T** the affected side.

d **F—** This is seen in lesions of the tibial (medial popliteal) nerve due to paralysis of the intrinsic muscles of the foot.

397 **Birth injuries involving the fifth and sixth cervical nerve roots of the brachial plexus:**

a Are known as Klumpke's palsy. ( )

b Are rarely followed by full recovery. ( )

c Are characterised by the arm being held in the pronated and internally rotated position. ( )

d Show weakness and wasting of the small muscles of the hand. ( )

398 **Following a peripheral nerve injury:**

a Loss of axon continuity is described as neuropraxia. ( )

b Due to gunshot wounds primary nerve repair is desirable. ( )

c Delayed suture is best performed one week after the injury. ( )

d Delayed suture is best performed three months after the injury. ( )

399 **After peripheral nerve section:**

a The axon grows distally at approximately 4 mm/day. ( )

b The growing end of the nerve can be localised by percussion. ( )

c Primary nerve suture should usually be undertaken. ( )

d The motor endplates degenerate after six weeks and resuture after this period is rarely satisfactory. ( )

400 **Brain tumours:**

a In the adult are most commonly glioblastomata multiforme. ( )

b In children are most commonly medulloblastomata. ( )

c Of childhood are most commonly found in the posterior cranial fossa. ( )

d Which arise extracerebrally are most commonly acoustic neuromata. ( )

a F-- This injury is known as Erb's palsy. Klumpke's palsy is a lesion involving the 8th cervical and 1st thoracic roots of the brachial plexus and is a rare complication of breech delivery.
b F— Full recovery is usual in this injury. It is essential to maintain passive movement and to splint the limb to prevent contractions during the recovery phase (recovery is unusual in Klumpke's palsy).
c T— The limb is also adducted and splinting should therefore maintain the limb abducted, externally rotated and supinated.
d F— This is characteristic of first thoracic nerve root injury.

a F— Neuropraxia is temporary impairment of nerve conduction. Loss of axon and nerve continuity are described as axontmesis and neurotmesis respectively.
b F— Primary nerve repair should only be considered in uncontaminated wounds.
c F— The optimal time of nerve repair is 3 to 4 weeks after the injury,
d F providing there is no local infection and the surrounding tissues have healed. The nerve ends can then be mobilised, trimmed of new fibrous tissue and carefully anastomosed.

a F— Although this rate has been described in experimental animals, in the clinical situation recovery rate is not more than 1 to 1.5mm/day.
b T— This is known as Tinnel's sign and refers to the paraesthesia produced over the growing nerve end in response to slight trauma.
c F— Except in the rare instances of clean division (e.g. accidental surgical division of the nerve) resuture is best left for about 3 weeks when the damaged area is clearly demarcated and local contamination has subsided.
d F— Motor endplate degeneration takes a number of months to occur.

a T— These are highly malignant showing rapid growth and marked invasiveness.
b T— These are by far the most common and together with other posterior
c T fossa tumours such as the cerebellar astrocytoma make up the vast majority of childhood intracranial tumours.
d F— Meningiomas are the commonest extracerebral tumour followed by acoustic neuromas and pituitary tumours.